After 29 weeks

A story of preterm wisdom for NICU parents

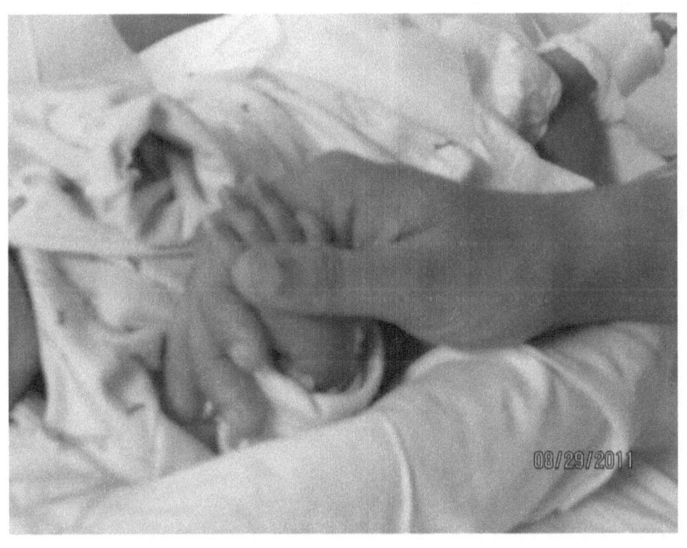

CHAPTERS

for Aarav,

for reinventing me at your birth, and every day after that. Knowing that you would read this book someday was the dream I held while writing it.

for Vineet, Neha, Mom and Dad,

for accepting me as a package, for loving me through it all, and for letting me choose a life that now resembles a playground, not a ladder. I would not be worthy of writing had I been on a ladder. Thank you!

introduction

This book is about my son Aarav and his preterm parents, Vineet and I.

Aarav was born on August 2, 2011, at 29 weeks of gestation, weighing just about 1.2 kilograms (two and a half pounds). He was cared for in the Neonatal Intensive Care Unit (NICU) for over 50 days, followed by a week in the hospital room. If someone had told me when he was born, that one day I would be worried about how fast he rides his bicycle, I would laugh and cry at the same time, disbelieving that my worries could be so small.

Vineet and I have come a long way since that day of his birth. Along this journey, especially the first 90 days of his life, we witnessed a life-transforming experience with an unprecedented share of learning, teamwork, and teeny tiny choices that were made for his well-being. I have always wanted to share the underlying wisdom we encountered with future parents, preterm or otherwise. However, my mind never let me get around to doing it. It got sucked into compulsions that I now realise were just meant to keep it busy. Three years later, as my heart and mind battled the choice of having a second child, my heart pushed me to write this book to silence the mind once and for all. The heart knows that such life-changing choices are not really mine to make, but I think somewhere inside it wishes that this story be written.

On a broader note, as a premie mom, I would have loved to read a book by another mother sharing her notes and experiences. A small tip, a word of caution, even an encouraging thought, anything that made me squeeze an extra drop of milk for my baby would have been priceless during those days. Every drop counts as you'll see. With this book, I'm sharing the little I learned, the little I observed, and the little areas where I was stubborn and hard-headed. Only because deep inside, I believed that all of this made a positive difference to my baby's health. I hope reading this will matter to you and your baby.

Wishing your baby health, happiness and love,
Anjali

a few things to note

I've intentionally left out names of doctors and medicines because names are not necessary to convey my message. Moreover, different practitioners have different approaches to preterm care, so I don't want to suggest one is better, instead tell you what happened in my specific case.

The health tips that I have included both for mother and baby are non-invasive, and based purely on my personal experience. I am not a doctor, and none of the material in this book is meant to be medical advice. Each body is different, and I request you to consult your body and your doctor before following any of my tips.

For simplicity, I have used the word **'premie'** to denote a preterm or premature baby, born before 32 weeks of gestation. I may use 'him' to refer to any baby, only because I have a son, although none of what I have written is specific to boys.

Some of the chapters, especially a few towards the second half of the book, have a lot more detail about the exact nature of care. I wanted to make sure that parents with a premie, or even friends helping a premie mother have enough pointers to apply to their situation. The remaining chapters are intended for all parents who may relate in different ways to my experience, and my hope is that everyone at some level

will connect to the spiritual lessons that I received in those
days.

"There are no ordinary moments."
-- *The Peaceful Warrior*

where the past makes its claim on the future

Tiny feet curled up on the hazy screen of the old black and white monitor. I jumped up, hoping to clutch the monitor with both hands. The ultrasonologist standing beside me resisted my movement, pressing her palm firmly on my arm, and readjusting that cold jelly that she had applied on my tummy.

"There's the baby. Very much inside."

An hour ago, her statement would have been a matter of fact. I was walking over to our sofa to pick up a book, without the slightest idea that within the next few seconds, everything about my pregnancy was going to change. It wasn't the quick walk to the sofa or the three floors of stairs I had climbed earlier that day. I climbed them every day. None of these actions was out of the ordinary for a healthy pregnancy. It was something else. Something from a long time ago, which was coming to make a claim on my body, and unfortunately on my baby.

More than 20 years ago, at the age of 12, I took out a little yellow notebook and scribbled a plan. Not a life plan. A plan to help me study for a bi-monthly test that was coming up at school. The timing of this test conflicted with a hockey tournament. I had also joined a dance class to learn the classical dance form called Bharatnatyam. With all this other stuff that I wanted to do, I was worried about failing the test. I was an average student and wanted to stay there. More importantly, I loved both sports and dancing and wished to enjoy my practice, rather than have this test nagging me all the time.

I had never made a plan before, so I put in some effort to ensure it would work. I scribbled days of the week, created time slots, and defined the exact subject and chapter I would study every day. I also carved out time for revisions and unanticipated distractions.

I loved making that plan. I loved the fact that I had boxed in this chore of studying into something easily doable, and had ensured that it did not interfere with the rest of my life. I gave myself a little check-mark every day when I finished studying. I loved following that short self-made plan. I told myself that if I had written something in that yellow notebook, it had to be done.

That first yellow page plan changed my approach to life. We won the hockey tournament, and I ranked in the top 10 students of my class on that test. Until that test, I was never noticed by teachers. I felt as if I had achieved something important, and it had happened because I had made a plan and stuck to it. It felt like finding a hidden key to unlock success, at least academic success. In my school, unfortunately, that was the only success that mattered. I went to one of those strict convent schools, where academics and discipline were both nurtured and applauded. Sports was provided for, amply so, but it was the academics that got the awards and the recognition.

For the next test, I made a better plan. It started early and finished early, with plenty of time to review my preparation. I did better, now among the top five of the class. The habit was reinforced. With academic success, sports and dance became extracurricular activities. I still loved both of them, but now I played to win and not to play. At the age of 16, I moved to another school, where sports, hockey and athletics, did not exist. I could not play anymore and was not inclined to learning a new sport from scratch. A year later, I met with an accident, broke a few bones and could not dance for six months. By the time I could dance again, my teacher had moved to another part of town. I stopped dancing.

Something else stopped too. My periods. Not completely stopped, but they started playing hide and seek, and disappeared every other month. Acne surfaced, leaving marks on my face. When I did bleed, it was irregular and heavy.

I did not worry about the periods. I was 18, and I always had some other goal to worry about and keep me busy. Academic success provided enough highs, and I had just met my future husband, so a lot was going on. I was making plans for every examination and sticking to them. As soon as I was done with one plan, it was time to make another. Life became all about planning ahead of time, ahead of the present moment, ahead of family activities, ahead of my own hobbies. I started worrying about outcomes. The past successes had somewhere created a belief that things were in my control. If they did not work out my way, it was because I was at fault, my plan was at fault. I stopped living in the now.

The heavy involvement of the mind in planning and worrying created a love for topics that explored the workings of the brain. Any practice that promised to teach how to control the mind had me hooked. I was drawn to spirituality, and debugging the mind became a hobby. I read several books, and during college breaks, I attended classes on Reiki, Art of Living, and other spiritual practices.

Heart-wise I was overly sensitive to criticism, especially from people whose opinion mattered to me. I was emotionally insecure and felt anxious when isolated. I needed someone around at home. This emotional pattern was probably a fallout of my early childhood, spent with nannies, when mom and dad were working hard to set up their business. Besides, I was confused about my future. Did I know if my plans would make me happy? In my world, things were black or white, part of my career or not, in my plan or not. I had not found my passion and did not know how to find it either. But I had got habituated to my plans and was scared of giving life a chance to plan for me.

What kept me going was my parents' joy on every achievement, and the security I felt in my relationship with Vineet. He was the opposite of me. Often in the present, in love with sports, and able to study for learning the concepts, and not for acing an examination. He was not fatigued by plans and outcomes. He was going with the flow, doing his best, and also staying open to the plans that life made for him.

Those were pre-Internet and pre-YouTube days. If you did not have an obvious passion that you could stand up for, you went along with what your parents endorsed. And that's how I chose engineering as my vocation, with a major in Computer Science, and graduated top of the class. When I look back on those decisions, I don't think they were wrong. But I do wonder if my academic success was a negative influence on my approach to decision-making. Doing well in an exam did not mean I wanted to work on that subject for life. I needed to do other things to figure out the base of a career. There was very little guidance. I lacked the support system that could frame my education in a broader context, and push me to try many things before I worked so hard on one thing.
Moreover, academic success is not great at teaching life lessons. I learnt the value of hard work and self-drive. But what happens when there is no defined syllabus or advance notice to plan? Was I prepared for life's real challenges?

The irregular periods continued through my twenties with bouts of acne, heavy bleeding, and hormonal imbalances. At age 24, I detected that I had Polycystic Ovarian Syndrome (PCOS), which is a common cause of irregular periods. A deep dive into my health patterns would later reveal that the PCOS developed after high school, soon after I stopped playing sports. Regular exercise had prevented the PCOS gene from surfacing earlier.

The PCOS got worse when I moved to the U.S., especially at business school, where processed food and refined carbohydrates were the most common food options for MBAs. The underlying insulin resistance, which is the cause of PCOS, was never addressed by gynaecologists, each telling me that PCOS is untreatable, and I should come back when I decide to have children. They suggested not postponing children for too long, but in my 20s, I could not appreciate such suggestions.

I met doctors only because I wanted to get rid of the acne, the migraines, and the recurring irregular periods. Although Vineet and I got married at the age of 27, our lives were dominated by our careers, our long-distance relationship, and our pursuits of higher education. The thought of having a child seemed further away than the moon.

One fine day, at the age of 32, the rewards of building new technology, moving to a new location, or pursuing a new startup failed to invoke the same level of enthusiasm in me as it had in the past. We had both managed to move together to Bangalore a year ago, and I searched for new meaning as we settled down to finally living in the same home. I wanted our new life together to feel more than our past accumulations. I wanted to focus my life on something more significant than each other. That's when it hit me, sort of suddenly, but deeply. I realised that I wanted to be a mother, and this possibility that had been buried away now felt inevitable.

A baby is born every two seconds in India. With the number of mothers I saw around me, I never thought of childbearing as risk-taking, nor did I see myself as particularly unique. Most of this pregnancy stuff seemed entirely predictable as per the media and the popular "What to expect when you're expecting" books. We were emotionally ready for the anticipated events, not for the outliers, that get mentioned in the footnotes of these books. Statistically, around 2% of births are preterm, and a small fraction of those are 29-week babies.

After six months of trying to get pregnant, based on our guesswork around when I would be ovulating, my doctor suggested mid-cycle follicular ultrasound scanning to monitor ovulation and gave me a tablet to stimulate the ovaries. A month later, I had conceived. Luckily because of the mid-cycle ultra-sound scanning, we knew when I would be ovulating, which helped us conceive sooner.

The way I found out I was pregnant was quite strange. I failed two home pregnancy tests, one of them on the period due date. I was in tears that evening at my doctor's clinic, and she suggested a blood test two days later, assuming my period does not show up. It did not, and the blood test was positive.

For the first few weeks, I behaved like one of those mothers that get portrayed in media articles. I bought all the books, started eating well and exercising, even playing pregnancy music to my little baby. I was blissfully happy, enjoying the idea of a baby growing inside me. Those days I was climbing three floors every day. We were renting the top floor of a cosy little house which did not have an elevator. When renting, we had loved the idea of climbing by design to stay fit. We also loved the elderly landlord couple who stayed on the ground floor. In hindsight, given my PCOS, it was a bad idea to stay there and climb three floors every day during the early weeks of my pregnancy.

One day, during week nine of pregnancy, I was walking over to the sofa to pick up my book, when I felt a surge of blood rushing out of me. I ran to the bathroom, and it gushed out even more. I had passed a large lump of something covered with a lot of blood, and I was horrified to think that I may have just passed out my baby. It was a fear like no other - when a dream is about to be shattered.

The PCOS that I had never fully addressed, the physical fitness level that I had never reached, the years that I had postponed marriage and children, the long-distance relationship that I had chosen while I pursued my startup and he pursued his Ph.D., the unwarranted stress that I had nurtured through the years, everything was coming back to make a claim on my pregnancy, on my baby.

That's how I landed up at the clinic of that ultrasonologist, with eyes shut tight, wondering if tiny feet will curl up on the monitor beside me.

I cried through my calls to Vineet and my mother, as I explained how I had passed that lump of blood. It had all the symptoms of a miscarriage as per my books. Vineet and I held hands all the way to the clinic. We had to wait an hour before the doctor could see us.

"There's the baby. Very much inside."

I was prescribed bed-rest for a week and house-arrest for two weeks. I was also given progesterone injections to keep the "uterus quiet". Those were my doctor's words.

Two weeks later, Vineet was traveling for work, and my sister Neha had come over. I was animatedly walking around the house while talking over the phone, and within minutes I felt that horrendous surge of blood gushing out. I was a nervous wreck, wondering if the baby could survive another episode. I didn't let the nurse move until she heard the baby's heartbeat, and even after some reassurance, I would insist she keep hearing it until the doctor checked on the ultrasound. I shut my eyes tight as I felt that cold jelly land on my stomach. I opened my eyes the very moment the doctor repeated the words I was praying to hear.

"There's the baby."

This time around, I blamed myself, assuming my walking around had triggered this bleed. Those around me assured me it was not so, and that my baby was a fighter. Little did we know that the real war was ahead of us, and he would have to fight his way through it all.

We started looking for a new home in a large apartment complex with elevators. For the next two weeks, as we searched and planned our move, I followed strict bed rest except when using the bathroom. Despite complete rest till week 14, I started steadily bleeding one night while sleeping. My doctor being on vacation, was unable to have me checked without formal hospital admission. I was admitted in the wee hours of the morning, and ended up staying two nights under observation. Since my doctor had strictly asked me not to climb stairs, Vineet and my father-in-law carried me on a chair to our car. I cried intermittently through that first night at the hospital, as the bleeding would not stop, and the nurse kept reassuring me that the baby's heartbeat was "normal". I hate it when the medical world uses the word "normal" to describe situations that would be unthinkable for "normal" people. Years later, another doctor would use words like "pregnancy wastage" to describe my episodes of bleeding. If thoughts could kill, he was dead. Once my doctor arrived, she sent me home, told me to rest and keep taking the progesterone. She was unable to diagnose why these bleeds were so intense and unpredictable.

Thankfully I did not bleed again, but I will never forget those moments of extreme anxiety followed by the most profound gratitude I've known. It's funny how nature had attached me to my baby right from conception. I already felt like I had a child, and losing him was unthinkable. While writing these words, I remembered an episode of the popular American T.V. series *Dr House M.D.* where Dr House kept referring to the unborn baby as a "fetus" and not as a baby. He assumed using the word fetus would undermine the mother's attachment, and she would not feel the pain of losing her baby. He attempted the impossible and failed, as any doctor would.

My doctor advised me to keep working from home, to worry less and keep myself busy. Luckily at that time, I was working on the early stages of testing a new product idea, and my colleague was a woman who agreed to come home for meetings. After five uneventful weeks of partial rest, I had another scan at week 20. I told the ultrasonologist that my doctor had explicitly requested for a cervical length assessment, to check if the cervical length was in the normal range. The sonologist was surprised and asked me if I had any previous deliveries. I said, "No, but I had some bleeding episodes in my first trimester". "Oh, that's normal, it happens." was her reply. Once again the unwarranted use of "normal".

The cervical length seemed okay, and I was told to resume regular activity, although nothing too strenuous. By now we had moved into our new home in a large apartment community, a five-minute walk from the hospital. It had a huge living room with beautiful French windows that opened into rows of eucalyptus and fruit trees. I was adamant that we find something better than our previous home. I was glad when we did. I wanted our baby to come into a home we loved, rather than something we had settled for in a hurry.

The trees attracted monkeys during summer, of course, we did not know that being new residents. One day a few monkeys opened our unlocked kitchen window and came in.

I was alone at home, and the last thing I expected to see in my kitchen was a monkey. I screamed, and my unexplained fear of all animals took over me. As I ran towards the bedroom to shut the door and call for help, I slipped and fell on the floor. Luckily I fell to the side, and not on my tummy. A few hours later, I was back again at my doctor's office having everything checked. She said she was having a monkey-week, because of all the mango trees in the area. Four pregnant patients had come in with similar stories. We later installed locks on all our windows, and that was the last time we saw monkeys inside our home.

Week 24 - I was back again for another scan. This time the cervical length assessment showed a much-shortened cervix, well on its way to shortening further. I had what doctors call "cervical incompetence" - the cervix starts opening up early in the pregnancy, because of the growing weight of the baby inside the uterus. This is not a common condition, and the reasons for it are unknown, but it is a very serious issue. If the opening of the cervix is not slowed down or halted, it can cause a rupture of the membranes and the birth of a premature baby. The doctor who named this problem with the words "incompetence" cannot be forgiven by a mother who has it, especially after knowing its implications on the baby.

We came home with a heavy heart. After enjoying four weeks of a somewhat healthy pregnancy, we were back to uncertainty, back to the cycle of fear and hope. Would this baby stay inside or come out any day? What would happen if the baby came out early? This time the anxiety was ongoing and very stressful.

I was now on complete bed rest, as gravity was my enemy. I was told to stay as flat as I could, so there is less pressure on the cervix as the baby gains weight. The only time I got up was to use the bathroom. Twenty four hours a day, I lay on a bed thinking about my baby. We had elevated the bed on the lower side so my feet would be a few inches above my body. I avoided having a shower bath every day. Vineet helped me with sponge baths during those weeks. He had to care for me like a home nurse would for an immobile patient. My doctor emphasised that week 28 was an important milestone in gestation. So every day from week 24 to week 28, we prayed to cross that milestone.

I would have driven myself crazy had it not been for a few blessings that kept my mind somewhat occupied. My younger sister Neha came to stay with me, so I had company when Vineet was at work. Vineet created a contraption of a slanting table, hanging in mid-air with ropes, that allowed me to type on the laptop while lying down. I googled and read every document I could find on cervical incompetence. I found a friend of a friend who lived in the U.S. who had the same condition a few years before me. She gave me more bed-rest tips and encouraged me to hang in there. I was grateful each night, knowing that my baby had stayed one more day inside the womb.

In week 28 of pregnancy, I was diagnosed with a urinary tract infection (UTI) and borderline gestational diabetes (G.I.), a result of PCOS and the ongoing bed-rest. The week 28 scan showed a very short cervix, 1.3 cm, and a one-kilogram baby inside. Vineet later told me that he cannot forget the worried look on the face of the senior ultrasonologist. She knew it was now a matter of days and not weeks. I was immediately admitted to the hospital for one night. My doctor gave me a steroidal medication that helped my baby's lungs develop faster. She said this would give my baby a better chance of survival if he were to come out early.

Two days later, at 10.30 pm, while resting at home, and watching a rerun of the movie Slumdog Millionaire, I felt a sharp pain. My water broke within seconds, medically termed as PROM - Premature rupture of membranes. Despite relaxants to prevent contractions, my body had decided that it was better for the baby to be outside rather than inside. After five hours of labour, with pushing and screaming, I vaginally delivered a tiny baby boy, weighing just about 1.2 kilograms, at 5.53 am on August 2, 2011, in week 29 of gestation.

My son Aarav came out crying. Vineet, who was convinced beyond doubt that we were having a girl, was speechless when he saw a boy in her place. For a brief minute, we both forgot that we had delivered so early. My doctor smiled to hear the little one cry at birth, and called him "boy in a hurry", although I knew he had no role in the "hurry" part.

That's how my story started. It started with my son Aarav's life of 29 weeks inside his mother and with his mother's life of 33 years that led to his birth.

I saw Aarav for precisely four seconds, after which he was whisked away to the neonatologist waiting for his arrival. It would be another 30 hours before I saw my son again.

Footnote: Tiny Lessons for Mothers

I did not know then, but I know now that doctors understand very little about the timing and markers for early birth. There is far too much ambiguity and conflict among doctors researchers and reality that mothers are better off listening to their own bodies and double-checking every symptom with their doctors. I know now that my body had a way of telling me what's happening inside. Still, due to a lack of prior experience, I was not equipped to listen to nor recognise those signs. It was my first pregnancy, and I had not read about nor imagined such possibilities.

I urge mothers to monitor their vaginal discharge right through pregnancy. That discharge is your best friend. Any change in volume or colour should be reported to the doctor so that possible complications can be diagnosed. My vaginal discharge had changed during week 20-24 and had I known the implications, I could have insisted that my doctor checks for cervical shortening much earlier.

I should have taken extra care to avoid infection. A shorter cervix implied the baby was closer to the outside world. Under-garments could be changed multiple times during the day to prevent infection, and vaginal washes could have helped too. Having extra Vitamin C could have boosted my immunity even further. I did none of these as they're not covered in typical books. I felt a contraction two days before Aarav's birth. I did not know then that it was a contraction, neither did my doctor warn me enough to assume any pain was a contraction. I should have gone to the hospital then, and taken the medicines that prevent labour. Since I went after my water broke, the medication had little effect.

where moms are marked fragile

The unwritten rule for all doctors and caregivers is to handle the mother of a premie with care, especially in the first few days after giving birth. Shield her from hearing negative possibilities, and don't share too much information, so she does not get stressed. Dads are also told to use their judgement before sharing the baby's condition with their wives.

A few minutes after Aarav was taken out of the delivery room in an incubator, Vineet had a briefing session with the neonatologist. A warm-up conversation to make him aware that he was now a dad of a 29-week old baby, and he should prepare himself mentally for what lay ahead.

"The next 60 days will have ups and downs. When babies are born so early, their health fluctuates, and many unpredictable situations do come up. Jaundice and a host of other issues are predictable, and all premies go through some of them so don't be alarmed when those happen. Right now, your baby seems to be doing okay, but the next 3 days are crucial and a matter of survival. It is still not clear how the baby will respond to being thrust out of the womb. He will have to learn to adapt to the outside world. Breathing is the key concern at this point, and I cannot give any assurances until a few days have passed. These will be trying times, so just hang in there."

To be fair, the doctor was honest, and he knew this was our first child, so we had no experience even with full-term babies, let alone a premie case. We had not read books, not heard of a NICU, nor did we have a remote family member who had experience with a premature baby. Doctors know the patterns, but each case is unique, so they never make promises.

I'm glad I was not given that talk. Vineet paraphrased some of it for me that night. However, his version talked about the baby being in safe hands, and how we did not have to worry about gravity pulling the baby out. Without an explicit induction, Vineet was now a member of the "Treat moms as fragile" club. I'll explain why this is important a little later.

As I lay in my hospital room, I was in a state of wonder and joy. The events of the night before, especially the process of natural birth felt as if I had connected to a larger source, where I was nature itself and not a mere witness to nature. Lying there, my idea of a NICU was a very quiet place with a warm and cosy incubator which replicates the womb perfectly and removes all the uncertainty, especially the force of gravity.

After a seven month pregnancy ridden with bed-rest, and a weekly shortening cervix, when going to pee felt like I was exposing my baby to gravity where he would fall out with the pee, this new phase was some relief, even though it lasted just a day. Somehow my doctor's constant reinforcement that I had to cross 28 weeks had helped me cross that milestone, which gave me something tiny to cheer about.

I was naive. I did not know anything about the NICU and what it meant for Aarav. The chance of taking home a healthy baby rises exponentially with every additional day inside the womb and improves dramatically after 32 weeks. I now know that the 28-week number was a better predictor of survival rates and not healthy baby rates. Everything was a probability plot at this stage. My baby can be an outlier on either side of the curve.

You would never know how tiny a premie baby can be until you've held one. When people say a baby was born small, they mean 4 pounds or 5 pounds and have no idea about 2-pound babies. I am talking about a baby that fits in the palm of your husband's hand. The tiniest sock or mitten needs to be folded in half and halved again before it can stay on the baby's foot. I had no idea myself, because the few seconds that I saw Aarav, he was all covered in fluids. I had never delivered a baby or seen a newborn up close, so I did not think much about his size at that moment.

I am glad I was naive and happy about that first day. It brings me to why I needed to be relaxed and treated as fragile - I could produce milk. Breast milk is vital for all babies, but it achieves a life-saving rather life-giving status for premies. Moms should stay as stress-free as possible because milk supply is highly correlated with stress levels. The more you're stressed, the less milk you'll have.

Around midnight that day, the nurse showed up with a breast pump, ready to teach me how to use it, and teach me to be disciplined about it. I hadn't realised that Aarav could not feed on me. I would have to squeeze out every drop I could get and send it to the NICU. She started talking to me with a clear call to action.

"I got a call from the NICU. They asked if the mom could squeeze some colostrum (first milk). They would like to give it to your baby in a few hours."

The new mother in me, also born at 5.53 am that morning fired upon hearing those words. I am going to give it my best and send those drops to him. I learnt with enthusiasm and pumped every few hours. Since I had had a vaginal preterm delivery, my body was prepared to produce some milk. Eventually, I did produce those few drops.

Footnotes:

Vineet was told to visit the hospital store and buy tiny steel containers. These are used for delivering milk to the NICU. We would eventually need 20 of these containers since milk produced at different times was not mixed. Premies are fed 12 times a day, so multiple containers are needed since moms cannot squeeze enough in one sitting. Later we shopped for branded air-tight containers meant specifically for breast milk. The NICU rejected these saying that they would like to ensure uniformity across babies irrespective of what their parents can afford. They mandated the cheaper, easier to boil, steel ones to ensure all parents can afford them.

As a mother of a premie, the most important investment you would make is a good quality breast pump with a generous set of accessories. We bought one from a store that delivered it to the hospital, so we had it the next day. You need to sterilise the equipment before each use, so it helps to have two sets of bottles and funnels. When in the hospital, you can use the hospital breast pump, but you have to ensure that the staff is quick to sterilise the funnel parts for pumping every 2 hours.

where babies are stronger than parents

I never fully understood why it was so 'bad' to have a premie until I walked into the NICU for the first time. With washed hands, dressed in a sterile green gown, I walked slowly, one small step at a time, my body still healing from the delivery wound and the small cut given by the doctor to protect Aarav's tiny head. It was a long walk, crossing two sets of doors, which finally opened into a large hall with bright lights, and ear-piercing alarms ringing all over. But I did not notice all of this then. My heart was racing, and emotions were bubbling up. It was the first time I was going to see my baby. Aarav was at the extreme end, and as I walked up to him, I passed many tiny babies all in different incubators with tubes and sensors all over their bodies. Aarav was in an open incubator, covered with many tubes and wires, his eyes taped shut, his skin dark and pale, and a bright U.V. light placed above his head. The name card on the incubator read, "Baby of Anjali, born on August 2, 29 weeks, male, 1.2 kg at birth." He was mine and every card and equipment assigned to him had my name. I remembered my mom once saying that in all of humanity, motherhood is the only relationship that cannot be questioned. I now understood what she meant.

For a moment I was stunned - I have never seen a human baby so tiny, almost under-developed, and I felt a sharp inner pain with the thought that I had given birth to this one - as if I had yanked him out when he was still forming inside. It was the truth, but I felt it then, only on seeing him. I will never wish any mom to feel that pain, ever.

He seemed tinier than the forty other babies around him, probably because he was the newest, and the others had been there long enough to gain some weight. Aarav had already lost weight - all babies do as they adapt to the outside world. Plus he had the added complexities of the zillion tests, brain scans, body scans, and blood draws that were carried out in the first three days of his birth.

I was not allowed to hold him that day. I could not see his eyes that day. I could not do anything a new mother dreams of doing when she finally sees her baby after a long pregnancy. Every visual I had nurtured through my pregnancy was not to be a reality today. I cried uncontrollably, every mom does on her first time with the baby. Even in that uncomfortable, unnerving setting, with alarms, babies, nurses and doctors all around me, I could not hold back my emotions. Tears flowed abundantly. The nurses did not intrude, until after some time one of them came and said, "he will be okay, don't worry". I could derive no comfort from her words. The only thought that came to me was "how could I put my baby through this!" He deserved to be held, cooed, hugged, and fed from his mom, not this plastic tube through his nose. If a billion dollars could make that happen, I swear I would have robbed a bank that day, but this was one of those many moments in life where the money is just a number in an account somewhere; it's not power, it's nothing.

Emotionally I was so broke that I ran out of prayers, and I also ran out of those bribes that I offer God when I feel desperate and helpless. Every option had been exhausted during the pregnancy, especially when I had begged the Universe to show me a baby on that ultrasound monitor. That was a pregnant mother's heart. The flood of tears had given way to a new heart, a new stronger one, a mom's heart. I was a real mother now. Strength came, and slowly it brought the realisation that this is our son now. Vineet and I are his caretakers for life. He needs us more than anything else, and he needs our spirit and our strength. We are now a family, not a pregnant couple. It was to be our collective mission to nurse him back to health. Every moment from now on will be about this mission. Taking Aarav home.

Mothers have a guidance meter, something inside that prevents them from getting depressed. I did not waste time questioning "Why Aarav? Why us? or even "What if ...What will happen?" I cried, said the Gayatri mantra in his ears and limped out, determined to pump milk and come back here to hold him through it all. Vineet was no different. Dads are the same inside. They sort out quickly what they have to do. They do more than take care of the baby - they also take care of the mom.

Many situations are unimaginable in our thoughts. When we hear of someone struggling through a loss, an illness, a divorce, an accident, we all wonder how they bear it, when our own systems seem to collapse at the very thought of such a possibility. If I had ever seen a NICU before pregnancy, I would not be able to convince myself to have a child. That's how fragile the mind can be. That's how fragile it can make us if we listen to it. The potential for facing life is all in the heart, and the mind has no clue how much strength we have inside. When needed, that strength comes. Trust me.

That was the second time in my life when that strength came to me. The first time was when I delivered Aarav. A year ago, I remembered reading a book on vaginal deliveries. I wanted to know why many women fear it at some level. Was there really something to fear, or was it something the mind fears? The author of that book said something very simple which I will paraphrase -

"The body is strong and also wise. It can bear an unimaginable amount of pain, but it is wise enough to know how much that pain should be. You need not worry nor try to guess for it. Just let your body lead. If your body decides that the pain is too much, it will send a signal, and you'll probably become unconscious, but until then don't worry. Push and breathe, and leave the pain management to the body".

That's why I never feared the delivery and my mind shut down entirely in labour. I hope somewhere this helped Aarav come out safely.

For the second time in life, I knew I had to follow this advice. I have to believe that Aarav's body is strong and wise. It will deploy his strongest survival instincts and will signal pain and cry for help when needed. I cannot do it for him, and I should not worry about it. Nature will take care of him. This is yet again time for heart and action, not for the mind or for its thoughts.

Footnotes: NICU rules

- Every Level 3 NICU may have slightly different rules, but most of them will want you to stick to a schedule to meet your child. Mothers were allowed from 8am to 11pm. Fathers were allowed only once a day for 30 minutes. This was brutal for Vineet. They wanted to minimise infections and wanted as few people as possible around the babies. No bras, no socks, no shoes, no sweaters allowed inside. Wash up and wear only a sterile gown before you enter.

- Every morning at 10.30am, we had a briefing with a neonatologist who gave us an update on the baby's progress. All 40 parents had to line up outside and meet the doctor before walking in. This ritual made us bond with other parents. We did not know each other's names, and we did not get a chance to speak to every single parent. But we still knew each parent in a way that recognises why we are here and feels we are in this together.

- Kangaroo Mother Care (known as KMC) is a practise now followed in most NICUs. It is a practice of keeping a naked premie baby directly on the mother's skin (near her heart) and being held warmly by the mother wrapped in a gown. This is an attempt to replicate the womb to help the baby grow and heal faster. Usually, KMC is allowed after a few days of observation. My advice to mothers is to keep asking the doctor for KMC every day until they relent, so you get to start KMC as soon as possible. I pestered my doctors, and they allowed me to start on day 3 with 30 mins each day and gradually allowed multiple sessions of an hour each. Beyond medical care, there is a bond that exists between a mother and a baby, and I witnessed how much both Aarav and I benefited from the KMC practice. It made me feel physically like a mother, and he was in supreme bliss to be out of that incubator and off those tubes and on my heart. It was as if he is back inside the womb. Fathers were also allowed to do the KMC ritual if the mother was not well.

• When in the NICU, I urge every parent to read all the posters and memorise the rules. Ask questions if there is any concern. Follow every rule or question it but never ignore it.

where nature brings nurture

Now it was time to produce the really sacred stuff - breast milk. I was emotionally shielded by all to do this job. I don't need to explain here why breast milk is sacred food. Many books will tell you that, but I do need to tell you it's true. For all babies, and especially for a preterm baby, there is no equal substitute. The only reason for not giving breast milk is the inability to produce milk due to a physical, emotional or medical reason. The protection elements and delicate balance of nutrients that nature makes is unmatched to this day by any man-made milk substitute. A baby's digestive system is not designed for anything else in those early weeks after birth.

The nurses in my hospital had ensured I was pumping from day one. I was following a daily rhythm of pumping alternate or both breasts every 2-3 hours. To say that it was difficult to produce milk without my baby sucking, or even his sheer presence in the room, would be an understatement. But I never complained because my part was so small compared to what Aarav was going through. I just had to show up and pump.

I was told to visualise my son, relax my body, and de-stress in any way I could, but some days were just hard. I produced more tears than milk in some pumping sessions. In the first few days, I managed 5-10 ml and that too with great effort.

That's about a teaspoon of milk which I promptly gave the NICU. Luckily Aarav's intake in those first few days was 2 to 4 ml every 2 hours.

Most books would tell you that breasts work on the demand and supply principle. However, without a baby sucking and demanding, that principle is out of balance. Pumps rarely work as well as they should, and don't create enough demand. I did everything that every mother on the Web recommended - breast massages, warm baths, eating fenugreek and other natural stimulants, etc. I even scheduled my pumping session just after Kangaroo care with Aarav, so I felt all mommy-like inside.

The NICU had a private area exclusively for mothers who wanted to pump milk during their visits. I tried it once but could not get myself to go there again. Our hospital reserved a few incubators for premies born to parents from low-income homes, who need level-3 NICU care, and not the one provided in government-run free hospitals. Such parents are unable to afford a level-3 NICU; hence this initiative is part of this private hospital's social responsibility. Once admitted inside the NICU, all babies, irrespective of where they come from are treated equally, and rightly so.

The waiting area was a shared space for all mothers. That one time that I ventured there, I found it heart-wrenching to see some of these mothers pumping milk either with bare hands or with a manual pump. They simply lacked the resources to buy the electric pumps. Also, because of their upbringing, they would first spend on conducting a pooja (prayer ceremony) for the baby's health rather than spend on their own comfort.

It was easy for me to believe that the hospital should have provided an electric pump in the pumping area, but I am sure the reuse and sterilisation aspects would impose infection risks. Moreover, every department in the hospital would want funds for other economically challenged patients. In a country like India, free health-care can become unsustainable unless the government helps you out. I was shaken by the herculean effort of those mothers to squeeze out milk without a good pump. I am sure they were in pain. Their eyes were shut tight. That experience underlined the realities of life and my own blessings in being able to afford the best pump.

Aarav's demand for milk grew slowly in week one and then doubled suddenly in week two. My supply started falling short. I panicked and voiced my fears to my doctor (neonatologist). I had seen the nurses supplement some babies with formula feeds so I thought I will let his doctor know I was falling short. His reply was sharp and clear -

"You have to pump. Go see a lactation expert if you need to but don't assume there is an option. I will not consider any formula substitutes for your baby until there is a risk of starvation."

I still cannot believe he used these words. He violated the rule of not stressing out the mother, but I know why he did it. The milk was more sacred to him than keeping me stress-free. He did not let my mind think there was a choice. I respect him for that. If he had probably been softer on me, it would have reduced my milk supply even further. I was now forced to think only of those options that increased my milk supply.

Those days I was sleeping 5 or 6 hours each night. I used to pump after 6 hours of sleep. That early morning session was my best in the day, almost two or three feeds worth of milk got produced. Premies are fed every 2 hours, so 12 feeds a day. Their tiny stomachs, along with the need to gain weight, requires this pattern to continue until they reach the original due date.]

Our body rests and recharges in sleep. Breasts also work the same way. Sleep works like magic for milk production. After being given that threat of starvation, I decided to use sleep to my advantage. I woke up every 3 hours even at night to pump milk. I pumped for 20 minutes at 3 am. My body believed that

Aarav was hungry again and produced a lot more milk. I now had two pumping sessions at night, where I got a lot more milk than in the day-time sessions. On some days, I had more than I needed which I froze for later use.

When Aarav's demand shot up again, I was able to give this frozen breast milk to the NICU. Although one of the other doctors was a little concerned and wanted fresh milk (pumped in last 24 hours), my baby's doctor was supportive. He knew I was doing the best I can. He had threatened me earlier. As long as I brought human milk and not cow's milk, I had his blessings.

On another note, moving our home was the best decision from a NICU point of view. We were a 5-minute walk from the hospital. I was saved the stress of a commute, and it allowed me to pump at home and not in the waiting rooms. It allowed me to eat at home, and make multiple trips to meet Aarav at any hour. Parents who lived far away had a tough time and spent a large part of their day either in commute or in the waiting room. Mothers had less time to pump each day, and the commute tired them out. Some couples rented a service apartment nearby, which was a smart idea.

Many weeks later, I bumped into one of the hospital dieticians in the elevator. I asked her for tips to increase milk supply - in that phase, I was asking everyone I met. She gave me a good tip, and I used it for a long time. She said milk is a liquid produced by the body, no different from urine. Apply the same principle that you apply for your kidneys.

"If you drink a lot of water very frequently, you will produce more milk. Drink 500ml of water every 2 hours, or drink lots of juices and soups."

It worked for me. I was surrounded by advice from older women who insisted that eating high-energy foods will produce more milk, given my weight was on the lower side, but actually drinking fluids worked better.

"You can't control everything. Sometimes you just need to relax and have faith that things will work out. Let go a little and just let life happen."

-- *Kody Keplinger*

where skipping beats is the only way to breathe

Aarav remained in that last row of babies at the NICU for the entire first week. On day 3 and 4, I noticed even tinier babies being brought in (week 28 or 27 deliveries). They took Aarav's original spot, and he moved to another position in the same row. That was the high-intensity area. Babies were ordered by the seriousness of their situation. Lower the age, higher the intensity of care.

It was strange how a tiny part of my heart took comfort in seeing smaller babies come in. Somewhere inside I thought that if they made it, Aarav could make it too. The mind can be stupid sometimes. Little did I realise that surviving was not the only concern of doctors; babies had to stay healthy without any long term complications, and each day less in the womb drastically affected the chance of normalcy. Birth at 34 weeks is considered as just about sufficient by the medical world.

Aarav was not on a ventilator. He was breathing on his own, and he continued to be under the U.V. light, which was a treatment for the jaundice he had developed. He also had a UTI (urinary tract infection), the cause of which was proving a little hard to nail down.

One night, that first week, I happened to show up late at 11 pm to deliver some pumped milk. The night feeds for 11pm, 1am, 3am, 5am, and 7am needed to be given in advance to avoid a trip at 3am. By now, I recognised most of the NICU staff, especially the nurses who took care of Aarav. My favourite nurse was on duty that night. There was something about her eyes that made me relax around her. She was getting his feed ready - making sure it was at room temperature. She sucked the milk from the container into a syringe and then pushed it through one end of the tube, located at his nose. The other end was in his tummy. The moment the milk touched the insides of his tummy, he opened his eyes for a few seconds. I saw his eyes for the first time that night. Dark greenish, half-closed, struggling to stay open. Seeing those eyes for the first time made me feel like he is a real person, ready to wake up and run to me. I wanted to pick him up in my arms, but my time was up. No moms after 11 pm.

As I wiped away a tear, I heard a squeaky sound - Aarav had the hiccups. His tiny body, with even smaller lungs, was pulsating up and down. It was hard to see. I wanted to make them stop. The nurse reassured me that hiccups are common, and would stop on their own. I kept insisting we should do something to stop them. She smiled and told me that hiccups were good for his lungs. Not again! That morning he cried when they removed the urine bag taped on him. When I tried to comfort him, the nurse told me that crying is good for his lungs. Babies that tiny don't cry from their throats, their entire body comes together to cry. You feel like a criminal for making them cry - they're so fragile that you can see their heart cringe in the effort to cry. So the claim that hiccups and crying are good for the lungs does not go down well with premie moms.

The nurse may have been right, but I was determined to make them stop. A few more minutes of hiccups followed. Eventually, the nurse told the junior doctor on duty to come over and calm both the mother and the baby. The junior doctor, probably trained under Aarav's chief doctor, used her trump card. She said I should be focusing on getting home and pumping milk as they'll need more soon. "Get some rest and let us take care of him". And finally the punch line - "We cannot have you fall sick over the next 2 months. Don't let small things stress you out." I felt like stabbing her for playing this card.

There were countable moments in my life when I had shut up and swallowed my emotions. Vineet will vouch for this. He has become accustomed to seeing me bombard the doctor with endless questions written carefully after pouring over medical papers or blogs. I had vowed not to do so this time. It would have freaked us out to read medical possibilities and their probabilities. I kept my word. I said the Gayatri mantra in Aarav's ear, turned back twice while walking down the hall to look at him, which was my subconscious superstitious ritual in the NICU, and left for home.

I wish I could say that I heard his hiccups as I kept walking down that hall. Even if I had been blessed with dog-hearing powers, that would be impossible. NICUs are the noisiest places on earth, and I'm not even exaggerating. Each baby is plugged into those ominous-looking monitors that produce wavy signals and counters. At any given point, one of the alarms connected to the 40 babies was going wild because the oxygen saturation, or the heart rate, or the body temperature, was not within normal limits. The red light above the machine was blinking, and the nurse was on her way over. Often it was a false alarm, produced because the signal dropped due to some movement by the baby, but it was so loud that one would never take a chance.

My Aarav slept in this place, a place without a millisecond of silence. I wondered if he would sleep at our quiet home, or would he find the silence too eery. Right to this day when I remember that part of my life, I can hear those alarms in some dark corner of my mind, a hidden corner that I never want to visit again, never again. God willing.

"Hope is a good thing, maybe the best of things, and no good thing ever dies."
--The Shawshank Redemption.

where nothing happens and that's a good thing

Talk to parents who have had a child spend a long time in the hospital, or have had a child with a chronic illness, or a lifelong condition that erupts once in a while. One thing they will all say is this - "We are thankful for days when nothing happens. Thankful that today is the same as yesterday and the same as the day before. We celebrate such days because we know that an eventless day is good for our children."

Vineet and I had entered this phase too. We visited the NICU four times a day, and each time we hoped no one would have any news to report to us. We had learnt that any news is always bad. The usual stuff - the tiny grams of weight gained, the feeds, the antibiotics for the UTI, the blood draws, or the jaundice was not news. We never wanted to be the parents who the doctors are waiting for, or who get that emergency call. The one time when the NICU did call Vineet (they call dads first), his heart skipped a beat or more before he answered the call. He muttered a meek 'hello'.

"Sir, the baby of Anjali will need more milk. Doctors have increased the feed. Can you bring some more within two hours?"

"Yes, Yes, Yes", relief and happiness evident in the number of yes-es he uttered.

As we prayed for routine days, we became overly sensitive and acutely aware of small changes in the facial expressions of our doctor. One morning, at the daily parent briefing session, the look on his face resembled that of someone having a moment of recall - as if he was saying to himself "Ah...the baby of Anjali case...I need to tell them now." I almost choked on my own breath and stared at him. He started talking, in as direct a tone as possible - "The baby has a small hole in his heart. All babies have it when they're inside the womb. It usually closes naturally over a few days after birth."

The word "hole" felt like he had dropped a bomb on my heart, but once he said "all babies have it" I recovered. He continued, "But (our hearts froze again on but) your baby's hole is larger than what we usually allow to close on its own. It's symptomatic."

My heart was saying - "You better not tell me that the medical world has not figured out how to close it!"

"There is a simple medicine to close it" Okay! So then?
"But due to his urinary tract infection and other blood parameters which are much higher than the normal range, we cannot give the medicine. We have to wait for this one blood parameter value to fall, and I think the infection is not letting it fall. We're repeating his urine cultures, and hoping to treat it quickly. I want to give the dose within the next 2-3 days. I

wanted to let you know that this issue is the main one I am focusing on, and we need to fix it soon. Right now, the baby seems fine even with the larger hole. We'll know if it starts to cause him a problem."

I did not want to hear the last part, although I knew he had some good reason to tell us. From that moment, onwards, that hole was the only thing that bounced around in my mind. I wanted to google every medical term he used when explaining the problem. I've left them out intentionally in this book. After that conversation, I crawled into the NICU, my body feeling as if a giant reptile was crawling all over my skin. I was not able to get myself to smile when I saw Aarav. Unable to hold in my anxiety, I approached my favourite nurse and asked her about this issue. She was officially not allowed to talk about my baby's case, but she said this issue happened to some babies and was fixed once the medicine was given. She listed ten other babies in the NICU at this moment who had high levels of that blood parameter, which she said was common in preterm babies. The only issue with Aarav was that we needed to bring this value down quickly because his heart required us to close that larger-than-normal hole. I slowly realised that I was talking to the wrong person, and in the wrong place - every baby here was the same as Aarav. Among the 100 things that could go wrong with premies, each baby here had developed at least 2 or 3 conditions and must fight through them to survive. Nurses saw the same issues all the time. They're used to this, but I am not "used to" hearing any of this.

A minute later, I was supposed to do KMC, hold my tiny baby's heart, on my heart, knowing his heart had a hole in it. How could my touch be healing when every cell in my body was shrinking with fear? I am not particularly weak, but using the words 'hole' and 'heart' in the same sentence will paralyse any mother, let alone an 8-day old mother of a 1 kg baby.

Vineet had his way of dealing with the stress. He started reading up on it on the Internet, read every article he could find. He was never the one among us to question the doctor's protocol, he just wanted to be prepared mentally if the situation needed him to do so.

My milk supply did not dip, but I could not sleep that night. I kept the night lamp on and stared endlessly at our window. We could see the lights of the tall hospital building through that window. I pictured Aarav's little face and his dark green eyes and prayed that our hearts would magically change places. It didn't seem like an impossible request. Not much to ask of God given the situation. It was my time to ask. If not now, when else? For all the talk about the uniqueness of each individual, I know mothers worldwide are the same. Every mother with a child in a difficult situation would pray in the same way. The world may classify each issue differently, based on length or severity, but a mom's heart knows no classification.

Another routine had set in over the next three days, where each visit we asked about the blood tests and whether the levels had fallen enough to give the medicine. The doctor wanted to give it early, but the levels did not dip. Meanwhile, Aarav's weight increased, and his feed was increased further. Every doctor seemed positive about Aarav's growth and resilience. Now that jaundice had healed, we were told to bring some real clothes for Aarav. We bought the premie size that's available only with select brands. Despite that, the nurses had to use surgical tape to half the size. Clearly, brands have a different definition of a premie size. We got him caps, mittens, socks and vests, washed with antiseptic liquid soap, ironed and delivered in neat Ziploc packets to the nurses each morning. Even a tiny doll wears larger clothes than Aarav wore at that time.

Every morning at 6 am the nurse oiled him, bathed him, and took his weight on a scale that was accurate to several decimal points. She then put his new clothes on him and got him ready for mom's visit at 9am. He seemed to be waiting for me. Now that he was in clothes, I felt a lot better about his health.

where giving feedback feels like playing with fire

NICUs and hospitals are no different from business-driven organizations. They're set up to manage tiny babies, with machines, processes and rules. They hope to meet their business goals along with their process goal, which is a healthy survival rate for preterm babies.

Like all systems in everyday life, the processes are not perfect. Not every nurse or doctor is comfortable with every button on every machine. Training is not perfect, either. Tiny mistakes happen every day. Patient feedback, although taken at a hospital level, is not taken when it comes to nurses or doctors or NICUs in particular. The strange thing about life is that we fill up a one-page long feedback form after dining at a fancy restaurant - did the waiter smile, was the food served hot, was the music just right, etc. etc. But when your child is 60 days in an ICU, no one is making you fill forms at all. Talking to the generic hospital feedback line or email address seems useless because, for the hospital, the NICU is yet another small department with a small number of patients.

Little things were missed, and we had no energy nor the mental bandwidth to complain. Gowns were old and torn in places. Chairs were few and uncomfortable for giving KMC. There was no seating area for parents even though doctors often arrived an hour late for the briefing. You could inform the head nurse about some of these issues, but you could never single out a careless nurse, or a junior doctor who was rude. It felt risky - like playing with fire. After all, my baby was 24/7 under their care. No human being, no matter how sincere, can be completely objective when dealing with critical personal feedback. I could not imagine Aarav surrounded by someone who had a point to prove against me, or even someone who did not like me because I reported something. I decided to keep quiet and let go of my usual tendency to give feedback.

Often when I went to the NICU, I observed the nurses writing furiously. They took extensive notes and recorded every pee, poo, medicine, feed, diaper change. I trusted that someone was watching over these notes. Sometimes I found a nurse so focused on finishing her reports for the day that she gave the feed 15 minutes late, and let Aarav cry for a bit. Sometimes I had to request her to stop writing, and help me adjust his position during KMC. Some nurses forgot to take the milk out of the refrigerator in advance of the feed time, and the milk was fed cold to the babies. Most often, they did not promptly turn off a false alarm because they knew the babies cannot complain about the noise level. They're sleeping right through it.

Every nurse was different. Some were methodical and diligent, despite the stressful nature of this job, yet others were less sincere. Some were happy to see mothers while others hated the fact that they're being watched. Only once I saw a nurse make a critical mistake. She gave Aarav an injection and forgot to immediately throw out the needle. The needle was lying on the corner of his bed. Luckily he could not move, but we were mortified when we saw it and alerted her immediately.

Every once in a while, we saw a senior doctor scolding a nurse or a junior doctor, and we took comfort in the fact that the bosses are keeping things in order 99% of the time. But was 99% enough when it's my baby? The fact that a level-3 NICU costs a fortune every day was not as important as the fact that Aarav was in here, and even one tiny mistake could be costly. I reflected on an incident a long time ago, when we got all worked up during a vacation when a hotel did not keep a promise they mentioned on their website and missed an important aspect of hospitality. Imagine how I felt when I saw a small error in an ICU, where I can't say something, nor can I just take my baby and go away. I chanted to myself to focus on all the good things they're doing for Aarav.

Facing a world of ICUs, where one mistake is life-changing, and knowing that human beings are prone to error, we need to elevate our faith to a higher level, where we trust that a universal force is in command and has the final word. Four times a day, Vineet and I reinforced this faith by chanting the Gayatri mantra in Aarav's ears. I've always had a soft corner for Buddha through my spiritual reading, so I also said a Buddhist mantra every day (Nam myoho renge kyo). Such rituals helped us close our eyes and talk to Aarav - "You're not alone in here my baby. Mum and Dad are not leaving you. We're right here, and we'll soon take you home."

The hospital had a Ganesh temple on the ground floor near the reception. The NICU was on the second floor. Each time I entered the hospital, I walked straight to the temple. Here I took off my shoes and prayed for Aarav's health. I've never been religious, always spiritual, but I had come to appreciate the power of rituals in reinforcing the spiritual. When I took off my shoes I wanted to signal to myself that I am not coming here as Anjali; the identity of my past years especially my education, my career, and my worth, had no relevance. I am coming unarmed, stripped of all identity barring one, that of a mother. With that one identity, I transcended my rational mind. I no longer needed to justify why an educated, liberated, non-religious mother is at this temple, investing precious minutes in prayer four times a day.

Over the years, I have realized that there are no rules for mothers - mindfulness, presence, religion, spirituality, logic, science, nothing.

A mother's heart and its need to express love are beyond all rules. I came to the temple as a mother - to share, to ask, to befriend a Force that knows it all, even though I knew that the Force was inside me and not in the temple.

The Ganesh idol in black stone had eyes that showed recognition to all who came forward. The fresh garlands and the unmissable smell of incense sticks made it easier for me to visualize taking Aarav home. Like his true devotees who knelt down barefoot on the floor, I knelt too each time; my new identity allowed me to strip away any social discomfort or embarrassment that often stops people from kneeling down in public places.

I know why the kneeling mattered. It stripped away one more layer of the ego, and I was that much closer to my true self. The sooner I get closer, the sooner I can quieten my mind, and ask for my prayers to be answered. This little ritual took five minutes, four times a day. Sometimes it took longer when I had to wait for other seekers to finish. I knew their prayers were important. We all gave each other space, we all understood. Every person passing by that temple in the reception hall knew why we were in front of God. They respected our need to complete our little rituals. Ten feet away, the security guard who had scanned my bags and seen the tiny boxes of breast milk knew too - "There goes a NICU mom, hope her baby gets well soon."

The unmistakable smell of an Indian hospital floor (smells of a powerful disinfectant), coupled with the scent of Ganesh's flowers and incense, infused with the subtle smell of freshly pumped breast milk. Senses were on a rollercoaster every morning, often interrupted by a touch of salt in a dropping tear. I guess the tears were necessary to complete the scene. To make it real.

where no one wants to go, ever

7.30pm. We entered the hospital. I prayed twice. There was an uneasiness that I could not place. We reached the NICU door. The female security guard gave us a nervous smile. "The doctor had asked me when you will be coming." Despite her sharp exterior and her dark blue uniform, she could not hide her nervousness.

My mind raced back to the morning visit when I had noticed that Aarav had been shifted out of the high-intensity back rows to the front rows of the hall. In this low-intensity area, babies were kept in closed incubators, and nurses wore white uniforms (to indicate they had less experience) instead of the dark blue ones that the high-intensity nurses wore just a few feet away. Seeing Aarav inside a closed incubator had made me uncomfortable. It was a complicated machine with too many buttons and controls. The nurses seemed unsure of all its different modes, and somehow, the chance of error seemed higher. The doctor assured me that a closed incubator reduced the chance of infection. However, my instinct told me Aarav was happier in an open one where the heat was not closing in on him. The feed had also been increased the same morning. Too many changes for one day. In hindsight, I should have questioned the doctors on why he should be moved to low-intensity when the heart issue was still unresolved.

Before I could think further about what happened in the morning, one of the stricter junior doctors came out of the double glass doors.

She spoke with measured pauses
 - "The baby was having some trouble with his breathing. He had puked out the feed this afternoon. His heart had raced to dangerous levels, and his condition became unstable very quickly. We've moved him back to the high-intensity area under the care of a very experienced nurse. We have repeated the blood tests and done some x-rays. The results will be here in 30 minutes. The heart is stable for now. Stay calm and wait for us to keep you informed through the night."

The last two lines seemed memorized. I tuned off the moment she uttered the word 'calm'. I don't know where my heart leapt to, but I remember not feeling it inside me. The mandatory hand washing, gown dressing was all a blur as we wobbled inside the NICU. Where was he? All babies look alike in that zone of the NICU - no clothes, only tubes and tapes. I was desperately looking at every station, trying to find him. Once again, my favourite nurse was there to guide me to Aarav.

He was Aarav, but not the Aarav I had seen this morning. Completely bare, with none of those premie clothes that made him look larger. His eyes were wide open, more awake than I have ever seen him, desperately trying to understand what is happening both inside and outside of him, and hoping something familiar shows up. Machines were beeping all around him, and I saw that they had pricked him and pained him for blood draws. "No KMC today Mumma?", my heart was speaking for him. Mumma had started crying. The nurse knew I would. She knew what had happened even more than I understood. She told me he was okay now, (stressing on now) and will be watched every minute. The chief doctor had been informed. He'll stay in constant touch.

The senior among the junior doctors came over. He had the blood test results. The value of that stubborn parameter had budged slightly. It was now at the borderline of what's acceptable to allow them to give medication to close the hole in Aarav's heart. They had concluded that the hole, along with the puking, may have caused the instability. They would keep his chest open and observe his breathing all night. They planned to give the first dose of the medicine that night. They would call us if needed. Please don't. I don't want to take that call.

We went home unable to make sense of what had happened, and what could happen that night. Vineet's parents had come last week to be with us, and take care of the home. I couldn't talk much to them or to anyone else. Vineet was much stronger. He had an unshaken belief that Aarav will pull through. He reminded me that our son is a fighter - a word he too had used through the pregnancy. I swung between moments of strength, worry and even blame. "I should have kept him inside. I should have never climbed stairs...." I knew this was my old weaker self which was talking, but I just had to let this tape run out. I had seen what Aarav was going through - the bare chest and wide-open eyes were all I visualized. If he can go through this, the least I can do is breathe through the night.

I walked around the house like a zombie. I finally sat in our bedroom and did the only thing I knew - pumped milk. At midnight, unable to sleep, I called the NICU. I asked to talk to Aarav's nurse. She assured me he was doing fine. The medicine had been given. The dose will be repeated tomorrow. Her voice was my saviour that night.

Since I could not sleep, my mind drifted to random thoughts. I pondered over the job of a NICU nurse. Does she ever get the feeling that "My job has no meaning"? The high intensity of the environment and the constant fear of a mistake must be exhausting. No cubicles, hardly any chairs, no fresh air, no unplanned breaks, and sticking needles and tubes into tiny babies all day. I thanked her for choosing this as her life's work. The work choices of so many people are responsible for Aarav's safety today. Their presence was more reassuring than anything I had pursued or piled up. I reflected on my life, and wondered what will make it matter? I wondered how people deal with loss and with ageing, and my guess is that after retirement, people see life more clearly. Decades of piling up, followed by a decade of reworking the pile, hoping it will mean something. I felt a void that night, and a need to define my legacy or at least work towards making something that will matter to Aarav.

My past flashed around in my thoughts. I should have lived in the present. I should have valued relationships and family more. I should have made more friends, or kept in better touch with old ones. In those moments, I decided that Aarav cannot come home to what I was - a person never in the 'present' moment. I have to change myself. Being present can be my biggest gift to him. A mother who is not restless, not bored, not judging, not craving, just living. Could this be my legacy?

Today his life's situation is teaching me to be present, tomorrow when he grows up, it would be my turn to teach him back.

Just come home, Aarav. For the first time, your mother is mindful today.

"Nothing ever happened in the past that can prevent you from being present now, and if the past can't prevent you from being present now, what power does it have?"

-- Eckhart Tolle

where the mind and heart become one

The sun that rose the next morning was the same as every other day. But to me, it felt different, like a brand new sun. Probably because something had changed within me. I cannot place a finger on it. I walked briskly to the hospital. The security desk scanned my bags. Lord Ganesh was there in all his glory. I removed my shoes and closed my eyes in prayer. I could not do the prayer I did every day. I could not ask for anything. I felt the presence of God, but the only thought that formed in my mind was - "I think I have said the same prayer ever since I got pregnant, and I've said it a million times since I gave birth. You've heard it enough. I don't want to ask anymore. I don't want to think anymore. I don't know what will happen. I just want to breathe."

So that's what I did. With my eyes closed, my mind drifted to my breath and stayed with it, and a few more breaths later, I was done. For the next 40 days that Aarav remained in the NICU, that's how I prayed. That's how I pray to this day. Saying a mantra is more of a habit now. My real prayer is just breathing in the presence of God.

The following day, once Aarav was stable, and being cared for by senior nurses in the high-intensity area, we decided to meet the head of the neonatal department. We questioned him on why Aarav had been shifted to the low-intensity area despite his heart issue being unresolved. The department head was defensive. We learnt that there was an overflow of just-born premies in the high-intensity area. He unknowingly revealed that there was some error by the less-experienced white-dressed nurse in the low-intensity area. Aarav became too warm in that closed incubator. Well, this senior doctor did not say this directly, but his entire defence was built around the fact that they have only a limited number of highly experienced nurses, and they have to reserve them for the newly arrived critical cases. "Sometimes, the other nurses make mistakes. We did our best given the situation, and your baby is now back in the high-intensity area."

I would never know the truth. No one revealed precisely what happened that made Aarav unstable. I know that every day many precious lives are lost because of human error, or overconfidence. That's the reality of any hospital, including the best hospitals in the world.

Aarav improved over the next few days, and slowly the medicines had an effect. The hole started closing, and the urine infection was removed. We focused on increasing feed, weight, and maintaining an infection-free stay. After the events of last week, Vineet and I welcomed a return to event-less days, where producing enough milk was the primary concern.

The most blissful parts of my day were the hour-long KMC sessions - when Aarav would be on my chest without any tubes or sensors. Babies that tiny are magical, their aura casting a spell on everyone around them. His body was so responsive that he curled up with every touch. His heart was beating twice as fast as mine. Within a few minutes of landing on my heart, he would fall into a deep sleep and enter a world very different from the world he would wake up to. I sang songs, whispered thoughts, told him how my day had been so far, what's happening at home, and when daddy would be there to meet him. It was like chatting with a tiny Buddha, at peace with everything, and yet needing his Mommy.

He howled each time the nurse pulled him away after an hour of Mom's touch. His body reacted violently to the separation. The mother-child connection is physiologically and deeply wired. I witnessed it every day, humbled by the power of nature. Both Aarav and I would shed some tears after KMC, and he would go back to his feed and sleep, as I would to my feed and pumping.

Vineet's time with Aarav being restricted was treasured by both of us. Although I sat there, I let Vineet have his time with his son. He would talk to him, take a picture, help the nurse change clothes, apply a cream to any dry skin, and try calling him different names. Among all the pet names that Vineet invented in those days, the one that's stuck around till today is "Gubi", which means chubby in my mother tongue Marathi. He was far from being anywhere close to chubby, but that's how Vineet wanted him to feel. Often the nurse would let Vineet pick him up and cuddle. Vineet would forewarn me - "Once Gubi is home, I'm doing all the KMC".

I was always the hyper one between us, but in the NICU it was clearly Vineet. Each time an alarm went off, he would jump around as if it was happening for the first time. If another parent sneezed inside the NICU, he would be furious about him not wearing a mask. His heart turned mushy and got used to being in an always-alert mode. To this day, I see Vineet over-protective of Aarav and repeating those hyper-reactions that have been subconsciously imprinted for life. His behaviour invites comments from friends, who observe his over-cautiousness, and his ability to forecast what/when/how something could hurt Aarav. Those who have seen Vineet's injury-ridden naughty childhood are shocked that a guy who believed in total experimentation as a child is so protective as a dad. I am the only person who has seen how this change happened. I'm okay with it. When you've seen your son stay in intensive care for that long, there will be side-effects, and you would do what it takes to keep him away from hospitals. At least one of a premie's parents is bound to become overprotective and alert. In our case, it was Vineet. This also explains why it took us a long time to stop checking on Aarav at night and letting him sleep on his own.

A week later Aarav was moved to an open incubator in the low-intensity area, this time for the right reasons. Aarav was growing a little every day and doing well. Being a breast-fed baby, his weight was not increasing as fast as the babies who were on formula. On some days his weight was up by 40 gms, and on other days he was down 20 gms. However, my growth as a mother was exponential, and every day I grew more confident in knowing what made my son happy. I was his voice in that noisy place, and over time my voice became stronger and decisive.

One morning, I saw that the doctor had shifted Aarav to a closed incubator. This time I spirited away, found the doctor and questioned the decision. He told me that closed ones offer better protection from infection. And as Aarav is close to reaching the 34-week milestone, (if he was inside me, this would have been my 34th week), they wanted him to gain weight and go home sooner. I was very clear in my head that Aarav preferred the open one. He seemed suffocated in the closed one and relieved to be out of there during KMC sessions. Of course, I could not say this to the doctor, so I told him that I feel stressed with the thought of him being in a closed one, given the last episode. I convinced him by saying that if Aarav were to come home, he would be in the open too, so it's best we keep him in an environment that is similar to home. The doctor did not push me. In the low-intensity area, it's the mother's call so I could decide. I chose to have him moved to an open incubator, and the nurse did the needful immediately.

To be honest, my mind wanted to go along with the doctor, but my heart took the decision. I wanted Aarav to be comfortable, and more than anything else I wanted every doctor passing by him to clearly see him in the open, and correct any error.

Finally, after 42 days of intensive care, Aarav had reached the milestone of 1.5 kg weight. In the womb, he would have reached this milestone within 10 more days. He had also crossed 34 weeks of gestation. Babies born after 34 weeks are not considered preterm. My doctor issued a series of tests related to eyes, ears and kidneys to rule out any long term issues, or developmental concerns.

Some tests were simple and conducted inside the NICU, but some needed him to go to a specific department. It was scary to see him being wheeled out of there (any outside trips were always in a closed incubator). I hated the tests that involved injecting a dye, or those that involved blood draws. Those were brutal, and he howled through the injections. I put on my brave Mommy face at first, but one look at the needle and I was a ball of nerves. I sent Vineet for one of the more painful tests. He later told me his eyes filled with tears, when he saw them pass a tiny tube through Aarav's urethra to his bladder. I don't like to think about the pain that Aarav went through in those days.

Once when my Dad was visiting, I tried sending him along with Vineet. Aarav had a test scheduled that day. My Dad excused himself and requested to wait in the room. He could not bear the thought of hearing Aarav howl. I had not seen this side of my Dad. During my childhood, Dad was the strong one, while my Mom hyper-ventilated around doctors. Given how tiny Aarav was, the thought of a painful medical procedure on those tiny organs was unnerving to all.

where little things become big milestones

Aarav reached 34 weeks. It was a big deal.

The doctor asked me to start breast-feeding to help Aarav suck rather than feed from a tube. It felt good to be finally told to do things like a real mom. I was happier for Aarav. For the last few weeks, I had seen the nurse give him her finger (wrapped in a sterilized glove), and he sucked on that while the actual feed went in through the tube. Babies don't need to be taught how to suck, they do it in the womb too. Like all babies, premies have that natural urge to suck and comfort themselves. Aarav wanted to suck so he used to latch on to anything near his mouth. The real joy of a tummy full of milk is in the sucking effort. It was his time to experience that joy.

To my surprise, the nurse told me that my first few days of breast-feeding trials would be on an empty breast - I had to pump out the milk before I saw Aarav. The idea was to have him practice and not feed him. They wanted to measure how much milk entered his tummy, so natural feeding was a no-no as it did not let them measure. Besides, he was so tiny that he had to build up his stamina to suck hard.

Experienced nurses were great teachers. One of them helped me hold and position Aarav correctly so that his neck and back are not strained. Although he was barely 1.5 kg, he latched on immediately and was a natural at sucking, as if programmed at birth. I felt more like his Mom than ever before. After all these weeks, I could finally imagine life without a pump.

Next, the doctor asked the nurse to teach me spoon-feeding, called palada feeding in Bangalore. Palada is a modified spoon-shaped container, sort of like Alladin's magic lamp, which makes it easier to create a flow of milk into the baby's mouth. Spoon-feeding is one of those things that looks really simple when the nurse does it. Hold the baby close to your body with one hand, and use the other hand to spoon-feed. Press the spoon a little firmly at the corner of his mouth, so he opens it. Push the milk on the tongue so his natural reaction would be to swallow it.

When I tried it, I could not get him to open his mouth at all. He resisted the very touch of a metal spoon. He spat out whatever little reached his lips. My theory for this is that he recognizes the smell of Mom, and knows she can feed him the real way, so he refused any spoon-feeding from me.

Aarav's doctor gave us no choice in the matter. We had to learn. Spoon feeding is considered a vital method to provide some extra and measured feed to a premie baby after he is sent home. This method is to be followed until the baby has reached 3.0 kg (healthy full-term baby weight). To put that in context, it was until we doubled Aarav's current weight.

Mothers are encouraged to follow a 30-minute feeding routine every 2 hours. 20 minutes of breast-feeding and 10 minutes of spoon-feeding. The goal is to give 10-15 ml of extra milk by spoon to ensure weight gain. Since 12 feeds would be tough on the Mom's health, doctors advice that dads should do one feed of only spoon-feeding so Mom can sleep for at least 4 hours. Of course, doctors pretend as if this practice is a walk in the park. The real problem with feeding a preterm baby is that he is accustomed to sleeping 20-22 hours a day. Their brain still thinks they are inside the womb, where they sleep all the time. It's impossible to wake them up for a feeding session. They won't even get up to breast-feed. They don't always cry when hungry because their sleep is so deep. No wonder the nurses use tubes to automatically feed the baby without involving his mouth. The tube goes straight to the stomach.

You may wonder about using a bottle - why a spoon of all things? Doctors know that bottle-feeding is easier, but they scare the daylights out of you if you hint at the idea of using a superior breast-simulating bottle. Bottles are prone to infection, and not designed for natural mouths. They never let a premie touch a bottle. They warn you with stories of moms who were unable to follow the feeding routine and used the bottle. In some cases, within a few weeks, the baby was back in the NICU with respiratory or infection issues. Flat steel spoons can be boiled and cleaned more thoroughly rather than bottles with complicated shapes and accessories.

My struggle with spoon-feeding continued. My doctor was precise,

"You have to be able to show me that you can feed the child on your own without a tube. As a doctor, I'm confident that Aarav is now healthy, and most of the premie issues are behind us. I will allow healthy premies to go home early, so they are 100% near their moms rather than in this place. But if you cannot feed him the same amount of milk that he gets here, I won't consider sending him home at all."

I gave my honest reply - "Doctor, he is asleep every time I try, and it's impossible to wake him up every 2 hours. I pick him up and nudge him, but he won't open his mouth. He is never starving since he is fed every 2 hours. Once he starts crying, he refuses the spoon and wants only the breast."

The doctor just grinned - "Routine must stay the same as NICU. 12 feeds per day. I don't want him to cry and lose energy over hunger."

By now, I was tired of repeating my concern - "How do I wake him up??" I almost cried with the thought of not being able to do this ever.

"Sing to him. He knows your voice from birth. You are his mother. You can wake him up with your voice. Nurses use tubes. They're not his Mom, so they can never wake him up."

I softened when I heard him say I should sing. That was so sweet. No doctor had elevated my status as a mother in such words before.

With watery eyes, I relented - "I'll try but can we please keep the tube on for a few days at home, just as a backup. I don't want to miss a feed. I can bring him to the hospital to change the tube."

He toughened. "That's not an option. Don't even think about it. Keep practising. Keep singing. When you're ready, we'll shift him to a hospital room, so you can be with him for 5 days, without the tube and without NICU nurses. Aarav goes home only after I monitor his weight gain without the tube."

No more arguments. This guy was dead serious. He made it feel like a mother's examination - are you fit enough to take home a premie? In the Western world, premies are kept in the NICU until they reach a much higher weight, but in India, doctors use their judgement to make a decision. They want the premies to be with their mothers as early as possible, as they know that a NICU cannot give that same level of touch and care.

This was the second time my doctor had threatened me. Last time he refused to give formula until Aarav starved. This time he was saying - "If you cannot wake him up and feed him, you're not yet ready to be a full-time mom."

I walked back to Aarav in tears. I knew I was doing my best, but all the singing, moving, blowing air in his ears was not helping. He needed more time to get used to the fact that he had to feed on his own. Not happening soon. At 1.6 kilos, a baby only knows that deep sleep.

where you're nervous inside and nervous outside

Vineet was doing much better than me at spoon-feeding. I believed Aarav knew daddy had no breasts. It was still a challenge to wake him up. The tube was our saviour, and we used it every alternate feed. I hated that damn tube the first time I saw it inside Aarav's nostril. Ironically now I wanted it there. Two days later, when Aarav was 1.6 kilograms (3.5 pounds), my doctor suggested we move him to a room. That will give us twelve feeding sessions to practice rather than six.

It was a big day for us. Aarav was coming out of the ICU after 50 days. I was nervous more than I was happy. It was strange how one can get comfortable with hospitals. The first person I called was my sister, Neha. She had been my support through the pregnancy, flying in at short notice, and taking care of me through the bed-rest. I wanted her to be the first to see Aarav. My parents were also with us that week. They had switched positions with my in-laws who had taken care of us through all the NICU days. My mother-in-law managed my kitchen and ensured I was well fed, while my father-in-law delivered milk containers to NICU in the wee hours of the morning. Our families had supported us all along, and we wanted them to take rest in turns. The critical phase was not yet over. Aarav was still a month away from his official due date - October 15th, 2011.

The nurses wheeled him out at 7pm and brought him to the 11th floor of the hospital. Our room was preheated and ready for him. No one expected him to be so tiny. The pictures we had taken in the NICU misrepresented his actual size. My Mom was anxious. She felt we should have let him stay in the NICU for a few more weeks. I believed that having a 24/7 Mom was better for him than a 24/7 nurse if the Mom could feed well.

All the other details that were followed at NICU care had been noted carefully. I had replicated them in the room. These included,
-    Making him sleep on an angle with head higher to ensure better breathing
-    Cushions on either side of him
-    Washed hands and usage of hand sanitizers as often as possible
-    Heated room with the temperature at 27-28 degrees Celcius

-    Oiling, wiping, sponging, diaper changing at defined timings
-    A notebook to keep a record of every feed and medicine that was given
-    Ensure that he passes urine 5 or 6 times a day. This is the best indicator of a well-fed premie.

Despite all my notes and preparation, the first night was a disaster. Aarav was sleeping soundly despite the sudden shift from noise to silence. On the other hand, his parents felt like they were catching a train. 2 hours is a very short gap. We had barely managed to feed him a quarter of his regular feed (8ml) through a spoon over 20 minutes of persistent trying, then begged the nurse to use the tube for the remaining milk. In the spare time, I pumped some milk, grabbed some dinner, sent the containers for sterilization, and it was time to wake him up again.

It's 11pm. This is our first time with him at this hour. I was suddenly thankful for all the days that he was with the nurses through the night. I remembered that my friends who had kids had warned me, that although I am eagerly waiting for him to come home, I should soak in as much sleep as possible while he was in the NICU. Once home, there is no break for years, until school!

It's midnight, and he refused to wake up for the feed. No sign of even parting his lips. The night nurse suggested I stick to breast-feeding. After some failed attempts, he finally got hungry and latched on. He was sucking so gently that we wondered if he was getting any milk. Breast-feeding was easy, like auto-pilot, but it would be useless if he wasn't getting any milk. Since his needs were very small compared to a regular full-size baby, it was hard for me to detect if my breasts were empty or full.

As he sucked, I kept wondering if this was working. What if he does not pass urine two hours later? What if his weight reduces with all this sucking effort? I remembered my doctor's face and wondered if he will fail me and send Aarav back to NICU. I massaged and squeezed my breasts, hoping some more drops will get into Aarav's mouth. He was fast asleep, and it had been 45 minutes since we started. It's a wonder how premies sleep through everything they do. When the nurse came back, she was shocked to see me still feeding.

"That's too long. You'll over-feed the baby."

Really! I hope you're right.

The next two feeds were 1am, and 3am. We were so exhausted that we opted for tube feeding. Thankfully I had some previously pumped milk. I wondered if I'll have enough milk for the morning. We probably got an hour of sleep that night. We had to wake him, change him, and check urine at every feed. The nurses did very little. They were not supposed to help until asked.

By now, it was clear that this was not sustainable. Vineet had to spoon-feed at least once so I can get some sleep, and help my body generate the milk. Vineet started telling stories to

Aarav, enacting dialogues, and adding sounds, so Aarav stays awake. Vineet hadn't prepared for story-telling a baby, so he did what came naturally to him. The first story he told him was of the movie 'Gladiator'. Russel Crowe would have fallen off his chair, listening to this version of the movie. After 45 minutes of action and drama, Aarav had swallowed 15ml of milk (that's about 3 teaspoons). We were far off from the 25ml mark. The tube was not coming off that day. My doctor smiled in the morning when he saw our plight. Try another day. The tube stays on was the only statement he made.

We sat down and drew up a plan, while the nurse gave Aarav a tube feed. My sister and Vineet would switch places at night, so each of them would get 4-5 hours of uninterrupted sleep. She would come in at 10pm, and leave at 3am. He would come in at 3am and leave at 9am. I could never thank my sister enough. She did this for a week.

I decided that I would religiously follow the doctor's timings rather than worry about Aarav being hungry. Only 20 minutes of breast-feeding, and 10 minutes of spoon attempts. The doctor assured us that if he gets less feed in one session, his body will make up in the following session. We'll know in 24 hours.

Now for the hard stuff. I was sure my singing was not going to wake him up. Are you kidding me, doctor? Those NICU alarms blaring in his ears never woke him up. My singing had no chance. I was jealous of those nurses - they had it easy, just push the milk into the tube. No sweat.

While venting my frustration aloud, it dawned on me that I was not the first Mom having this problem. I listed three moms who I had made friends with over the last 50 days of daily visits. We had discussed weight issues and pumping troubles. They had graduated and taken their babies home last week. How did they pass this test?

I called them immediately. One of them had been struggling with breast-feeding, as her baby girl had refused to latch on. Her baby was receptive to a spoon, but since the feed had increased, she was using a special bottle. She hadn't told the doctor. Her baby was hungrier than Aarav because spoons never gave a full feed. One trick she used to wake up the baby was to remove the layers of clothing, so the baby feels cold. Ten minutes before feed time, she would remove all the layers and wait for the baby to wake up.

Worth a shot, although it felt a little harsh. I increased the heat only slightly and removed Aarav's covers as instructed. He fidgeted for a few minutes, and gave a small cry, enough for my sister to quickly pick him up and land him on me for the feed. In that semi-awake state, he sucked for 20 minutes and fell asleep. He refused the spoon, but at least we were now quick at waking him up.

Here's the routine - Clothes off. Wake up. Left breast. Cover up. Sleep off. Put down. 2 hours later repeat with the right breast.

After 8 such feeds, Aarav had maintained his weight at 1.66 kg and passed enough urine. His doctor was happy, but he warned me that exclusive breast-feeding was not sustainable with 12 feeds a day. I had to get more sleep. I was on a motherhood high, so I pulled off another day with the same routine. I was happy that I was having enough milk, feeding him straight from the source, no chance of infection, and the milk was always at the right temperature. No pumping, no formula, no sterilization worries. My life seemed better this way.

Aarav was on a lot of supplements - zinc, iron, calcium and a few others for lung strengthening. In the few hours that he was awake, we gave the medicines through a spoon. Some of them were disgusting, and he often puked out his milk with the medication. The doctor suggested we give the medication 20 minutes before a feed. Doctors forget that we need to sleep!

By now Vineet had graduated to better stories. Gladiator was replaced by the Jungle Book, Lion King, and Finding Nemo. He managed a half feed of 15 ml with one of these stories. His joy on reaching 15ml was a pleasure to watch. I had never seen this side of my husband. He did everything else - cleaned the poo, changed the diaper, wrote the log, and gave the meds. I just focused on the breast-feeding. Vineet was like a guard, checking off on all other duties.

Here's an example of his feed log:
9am| Left Breast - 20 Mins | Spoon-none|Diaper changed |
Urine
Yes | Stool No | Calcium Yes | Puke No|

His habit of recording every feed was very helpful. Over the next 90 days, we had filled up an entire notebook. When Vineet was at work, I had to write the log or text him what had happened so his records would be complete. At some point, he migrated the log to his phone, so it was searchable.

Aarav literally had two moms once Vineet was home from work. Till today Aarav does not feel that Dad is a basic-feature version of Mom. Dad is fully loaded with everything except the milk. On many days, Mom was tired, or acidic, or just sleep-deprived, but Dad was ON. I was a mess without sleep, but Vineet's body was used to surviving for days on very little sleep. His five years of graduate student life during his PhD had trained him well for a premie child. It took me a while (almost 9 months) before I was able to go back to work, and then too, I was on antacids for many weeks due to sleep issues.

I had never thought Vineet would be so into his baby. Looking back, it should not have surprised me. He had himself grown up with a very hands-on father who helped with homework and housework. I had known Vineet since college, and right through our relationship Vineet had always been a person who loved kids and held this firm conviction that he would be a great dad someday. It's a strange feeling when you actually see a side of your husband that he has been reserving only for his child. I was a little jealous.

Those moments helped me understand that every person has a tremendous potential to love. In moments of crisis or fear, that love comes together. Although we never want those crucibles of life, we are grateful for what they make of us. Our teamwork in those days holds a special place in our relationship. We were not unique. All relationships have some phases of extreme teamwork and bonding. Parents are made to be at their absolute best when their child needs care. It was just happening all too soon for me to absorb.

The only vivid memory I have from those days is one where I am looking at Vineet trying three different types of spoons, all the while making funny noises and feeding Aarav. I remember thinking to myself that if I ever gather the courage to have another child, I will look forward to seeing this side of Vineet again. On all other days, the second child was unimaginable given what we had been through.

where poops play peek-a-boo

We were going through our notes for days 1, 2 and 3 when it struck us that Aarav had not pooped at all. Is that normal? He pooped every day in the NICU, so why not in the hospital room?

The doctor showed no concern. The NICU added some extra nutrition to the breast milk, which is often not digested fully. Breast milk is 90% absorbed with very little waste. Some exclusively breast-fed babies don't poop for many days. Aarav could be one of them. We were told to wait for 5 days.

Although we had not used Aarav's feeding tube for the last 18 hours, it still had to be changed. I decided that it would be the last tube change and we'll take it off completely if I could survive one more day without the tube. In the NICU, tubes were changed at 6am before moms could come inside. You never want a mom to watch this procedure. Babies howled through it. In the room, I told Vineet to accompany Aarav and the nurse. Watching a new tube go from nostril to tummy was enough motivation for Vineet to resolve that this tube would be the last one. It must have been annoying for Aarav to have this tube around 24/7, especially now that he was feeding on his own strength. We practised how to give the meds without the tube, and felt more confident with every rehearsal.

I wish I had better words to describe how it felt to remove the tube. Aarav looked like a different child. Happy and free. For the first time in his eight weeks of existence on this planet, he was without any medical stuff attached to him. That's the way he should have been brought to me after birth. If destiny had stuck to my due date, he was still to be born. But those statistics did not matter anymore. I thought about how far we had come. He was a real baby now.

Coincidentally, that same day a child development expert visited me in the hospital room. I had seen her weekly in the NICU. Until then, my questions to her had revolved around simple and short-term stuff - does the high noise level affect him, would he adjust to home, etc. However, now I was thinking long term, of the person Aarav would become. What would be the long term consequences of the pain he has been through at this premie stage? Would his subconscious mind have deep imprints of those needles and pricks? Would he remember all this in some unidentifiable way? Would it affect his temperament?

She seemed surprised. She was rarely asked such questions at this stage when the baby was still very tiny. She hesitated for a few seconds, before explaining to me that she does not think this will matter in the long run. Neither has she seen evidence of preterm pain having long term implications.

"This is too early for his mind to remember anything. Even with a full-term baby, there are so many experiences in early childhood that one cannot deduce the long term from the short term."

There is a lot of debate on what parts of a child's reactions and overall personality are a result of nurture versus nature. No one really knows the exact split. For now, I decided to let it be. I went back to worrying about the missing poop.

Aarav was cranky the next morning. We tried everything, but he was just not himself. I thought it was the poop issue. It had been 4 days since his last poop. Seeing me stress over it was not helping anyone. Finally, my doctor intervened, "If you are so worried about it, we'll make him poop. Nurse, please show the mother how to give the baby half a pediatric sized suppository."

The expression on my face needed no words, "Are you serious? A premie getting a suppository! He cannot even move, and I am going to make him wiggle with some irritating gel up his ass!"

That's what they do when babies don't poop. As long as the poop that comes out after 7 days is soft, we could be sure that he is not constipated.

"As a mother, you can decide to give him a suppository every 4 or 5 days if that makes you more comfortable."

He was cranky for sure, so I wanted to rule out the poop issue. Even a quarter size pediatric suppository is enough for premie babies. Aarav smiled when it went in, but once the irritation started, he was all red-faced and crying until it was out.

I thought to myself - Was life testing me or testing Aarav? Poor kid. Now he was crying even to poop. Hadn't we seen enough other reasons that made him uncomfortable? I was angry about the situation. Luckily his poop was soft as ever, and within a few minutes he was hungry. He had his feed and slept as if there was never a reason to cry in this world. This is the part about babies that I find absolutely unbelievable and so damn lovable.

On a broader note, the zero-resistance 'surrender' to God that people seek in books, in gurus, in religions, and in prayers was right there in front of my eyes. I cannot imagine a surrender as absolute, as complete, and as loving as that of a baby to his mother.

The new mother inside me was nervous about making mistakes. Did I do the right thing by pushing in that suppository? I was the one deciding and executing every moment of his life. As hard as I tried, I could never be perfect. Sometimes his bath water was a little too warm, sometimes his diaper was little too big, sometimes as I tried to burp him, the food that he had sucked with so much energy came flying out. Yet, he never complained. He just cooed, giggled, cried or responded with love, through all of this, his faith in his Mommy unshaken. I had nothing to prove with him, and his touch assured me that I was doing my best. The past moment or the one about to come did not prejudice his faith. His surrender to me stayed untouched.

I realized then that this is probably the closest I am going to get to understanding the miracle of life, of happiness, and the surrender that life expected of me. I have so much to learn from my baby, my tiny Buddha.

And yet, despite all my shortcomings, I was the one who got to play Buddha's Mommy. Surreal!

That evening I told Vineet that I am feeling very strong. Aarav's faith in me is powering my strength, and no matter what, I am always going to be the best Mom. Aarav is programmed by God to make sure I am that way. Vineet doesn't always pay attention when I get too abstract or spiritual. He probably only heard the words "best mom", and spontaneously replied - "Yeah, you will be a great mom. But I am going to be the best Dad ever!"

Okay, partner. That too is by God's design.

where doctors are not God just human

My Mom and sister were hard at work, getting our home ready for Aarav. My Mom is at her absolute best when it comes to cleaning a place, and making it baby-ready was her forte. She picked one of our bedrooms to be Aarav's exclusive room. He was 1.7 kg, and he would stay in that room until he became 3 kg. The home was cleaned to the pixel. Every curtain washed and ironed before his arrival.

We set up a white inclined board in the centre of our king-sized bed and covered it with a baby mattress. That ensured that Aarav will sleep at an angle. A heater was set up in Aarav's room.

New t-shirts were bought for my domestic help so that she would be wearing clothes washed in our home. All visitors, including family, had to wash their hands and feet before walking around. I did not allow anyone other than close family to touch Aarav for a whole month (until he reached his due date). Infection was the No. 1 enemy of premie babies, and I had heard enough horror stories to create a lifetime of fear.

By Day 5, the hospital room was getting on my nerves. I was lucky to be eating home food - my Mom sent it with my Dad every day, but I still wanted to be home now.

Aarav's tests were done, and the tube was off. We were in high spirits that morning, assuming that our doctor would give us discharge that day. He had another plan. He wanted us to stay another day. He did not have a great reason for doing so. We asked, and all he said was "give it another day". I was not convinced, but we obliged. I later felt he was buying time to prepare Aarav's lengthy discharge report summarizing the last two months of hospital stay. All bills had to be handed over to us, including the cost for every diaper they had used in the NICU. His junior doctors were probably swamped with other discharges and had not done their homework.

This brings me to an important part of our journey. The relationship between the doctor and his patient. Who was the patient here, and how should that relationship be understood?

The doctor always considers the baby to be the patient and not the parent. Unlike other specialities of medicines, where you communicate with the patient, in neonatology (premie baby care), the patient cannot communicate and is sleeping all day. The doctor sees his patient twice a day during his rounds. The parent is the entity who needs to be communicated with, but that is more a need of the parent and not of the doctor. All feedback about how the baby is doing is collected using bio-signals - blood, urine, heart rate, temperature. Doctors don't need parents to tell them anything. I almost felt that neonatologists are happy in this situation where they have such a non-interfering, non-judgemental, and completely trusting patient (the baby). Doctors are aware that parents are very sensitive, so they talk to parents about actionable stuff - feed, medicines, germs.

Our doctor is great with kids. He is known in the city for his ability to quickly earn the trust of any child at any age, especially those kids who hate most other doctors. However, he is a man of few words, often very few words. Other than a handful of conversations which I have described earlier, he rarely spoke more than a few words when we met him. On most days, his answers were two or three words.

His wife is my gynaecologist, and she had kept in touch with Aarav's progress through her husband.

I met her once, a few weeks after my delivery for a routine checkup. She is a bubbly and energetic person. Just seeing her made me so happy that I started blabbering away on everything and anything. I told her how much I hated the NICU, and that she should have scared me enough so Aarav would have stayed inside longer. I told her that one of my gripes with the NICU is that those neonatologists, including her husband, don't talk much. Their replies are too measured. She laughed and told me to just focus on getting out of there.

India is full of contradictions when it comes to doctors. The incentive setup is all messed up, yet the culture of the people elevates the doctor to a God-like status. The famous doctors have very little time for questions. Our huge population ensures that doctors have tons of experience, and see more cases per day than a doctor in a less populated country would see in a week. The good ones know the right answer, and sometimes make unorthodox decisions based on their vast experience. But their lack of time does not allow them to make you understand their line of treatment, or forge a deeper communication with the patient. They rarely touch upon lifestyle-related issues, although they know that the body works as a whole, and not as a sum of its parts.

I have been infamous for asking more than my fair share of questions. I often reject doctors who don't let me ask enough and stick to the more accommodative ones. In Aarav's case, his doctor answered my questions but kept the answers direct and short.

Here are some examples:

Would you repeat Aarav's heart ultrasound? I need to know
that the hole has closed.
"I don't need to see it. It will close gradually. If you need it, we
can repeat it."

For one of the tests, where Aarav was exposed twice to nuclear
radiology, I asked - "Radiation is supposed to be harmful.
What is the side effect?"

"It's equal to sunlight. Nothing more."

Aarav's eyes were watering and seemed to be irritated in some
way.
"Apply a few drops of breast milk." No further explanation.

I understand that detailed answers are complicated, and
doctors would prefer that the patient trust them because
explaining is cumbersome and lengthy. But I always feel that
doctors study more about cure than about health. Their study
begins when something terrible happens, and that's why I
prefer to ask some lateral questions about health and side-
effects.

I don't blame doctors. To the contrary, I hold them in high
regard. My baby is home today because they exist. They put in
the hours of grind required to be a doctor in India, where it is
a gruelling job in the early years, with low pay and poor
infrastructure. I have enormous respect for the profession

because they solve real problems, rather than work on making people buy more stuff, or click more ads.

The NICU stay made me regret my vocation. If I had to study as hard as I did, I should have got some hard skills that matter to this world.

It was our last day at the hospital. I was on my last question to our doctor, at least the last one for this week.
“Aarav is still cranky. The pooping helped a bit, but he was crying again later. What should I do?”

My doctor was his usual self. His eyes were focused on his patient and not on me. He had mastered the art of moving the chatter of parents into the background and keeping the child in focus. He checked Aarav's vitals, then turned him around, played with his soft hair, even amused Aarav with the giraffe toy hanging on his stethoscope, while I continued describing my baby's cranky behaviour. Finally, this man of few words said - "I think Aarav needs to be held. You're too stressed about the feeding. Just hold him and play."

I was speechless. I had not expected that reply. I guess my doctor wanted us to relax, and not be so worried around Aarav. He wanted us to play with our baby, rather than treat him like a fragile premie all the time.

The doctor then turned to talk to Aarav, his patient: "Ready to go home. I'll see you next week at my office."

As he walked out, he turned to me and said - "One last thing. Don't use that Johnsons' baby oil that I see on your shelf here. Stick to virgin coconut oil or virgin olive oil for Aarav's massages."

when a haircut turned into a nightmare

At 7pm, we drove out of the hospital in our little red car, Aarav in my arms. For the first time in his life, Aarav saw the colours and buzz on India's roads, as the city of Bangalore welcomed him with her trademark showers.

My sister had put up a little poster outside our door, "Welcome Gubi". It felt great to be home. Phase 1 was officially over.

Phase 2 involved the same routine. 12 feeds a day, 4 meds a day, and a zero infection lifestyle. We wanted to break that all-consuming cycle of fear and hope, one that had become our default over the last two months. We knew it would take a few more months. We had seen and heard enough baby cases, many with a sad ending, where infection strikes at home, especially cases of pneumonia and virals.
We had to be always on our toes, more so at home. There were times when our relatives labelled our vigilance as "overprotective", but I think the word "over" is meaningless for premie parents. How can we draw that line in Aarav's case?

The first night was daunting. Not being in a hospital, not being a few steps away from a doctor was scary. The "What if he was not ready for home" question popped up every time he cried. His feeding was irregular. He was not very comfortable on that first night.

The following day was a little better. His room was bright and sunny, and he slept most of the day. My Dad and sister decided to fly back in two days, and Mom would stay another week. The thought of family leaving brought anxiety. We were not fully adjusted to the idea of being just the three of us.

My mind quickly listed a few urgent errands that needed to be done while I had extra hands at home. My sister had spent many nights at the hospital and was comfortable managing Aarav for a few hours. Most of the errands could be done by Mom and Dad. One chore that I had postponed for several months was a simple haircut. I sport a short, low-maintenance hairstyle, which I used to trim every 6 weeks. I had put up with unruly hair over my shoulders for the last several months since the bed-rest prevented me from having haircuts during pregnancy, and the NICU life did not leave mind-space for a haircut. I resembled a castaway, with no access to salons. I figured I should cut it extra short, so it does not bother Aarav when I hold him over my shoulders.

It was a reasonable idea - get a haircut, nothing complicated. Little did I know that it would turn out to be the stupidest thing I ever did.

That first week at home, I was surviving on very little sleep, as Aarav was still adjusting. I was awake most of the time, and even when I managed to catch some sleep, I had to get up every 1.5 hrs for the next feed. My body's supply of breast milk must have fallen drastically, but I had no way of knowing. Aarav sucked for 20 minutes, and I did not realize he was getting less milk, especially in the evenings (5pm to 9pm) when my energy and milk supply was at its lowest. (It took me a while to figure this out. At first, I thought he had colic in the evenings.)

The following day, after feeding him for 30 minutes, I planned a quick haircut at 7pm at a nearby salon. I thought I had things under control. For backup, I had given frozen pumped milk to my sister in case Aarav woke up early. Vineet would drive me, so I don't waste time parking. The drive was about 7 minutes, and we would be back home in 45 minutes. Enough time considering that the next feed was 2 hours away.

I was so wrong. I'm in tears thinking about that day. Within 20 minutes of us leaving, Aarav was up and crying. He was hungry and tired. He had not got enough milk in that evening feed. In hindsight, he had probably slept off due to sheer exhaustion.

Initially, my sister tried to walk him, shush him, comfort him, sing to him, but he would not stop crying. Finally, she called me. I was halfway done, the left side remaining. I told her to try spoon-feeding and check if he is hungry. I told my hairstylist to hurry, and cut both sides to the same length as quickly as possible. My sister hung up and tried the spoon. Of course, he never took the spoon when hungry. He spat it out and continued to howl. My mother and sister were in tears watching a baby so tiny crying uncontrollably. My Mom knew it had to be hunger and ordered me to come home. I could hear his cries over the phone. Two more swift cuts to barely equal the length, and I was out of that chair. It was the worst hair cut of my life, and I was so mad at myself for stepping out that I could have pulled out my remaining hair too.

We drove back as fast as we could. All the way back, we knew Aarav was howling away. His only source of food was nowhere to be seen, and he was losing energy, whatever little he had. I started crying when I heard his howls of hunger. My Mom was mad at me too. He sucked like the hungriest kid on earth. I never want to see that kind of hunger again.

My sister took a while to emotionally recover from that day. She was the younger one and had not managed such a situation - a howling hungry baby, and no mother to feed. I swore never to step out until he was old enough to feed on a backup bottle of milk. It took us a few days to forget and forgive ourselves. Aarav was back to his blissful state within a few minutes of feeding. His *Mumma* was still the best, all her failings were unlabeled in his gentle ever-accepting eyes.

Every mother has her moments in those early days where she feels she has qualified for the "worst mom ever" title. I felt the same, and over the years, I found out that I was not alone. Other moms told me their stories, rather their nightmares. One of my friends had a similar story when she stepped out to buy pizza for her elder child who was throwing a tantrum. Another mum had accidentally dropped her baby from a low cot - the Mom was sleep deprived for many days and was breast-feeding lying down. Unknowingly, she had put the baby on the outer side of the bed. Luckily the baby was fine after the fall, but the Mom cried all night.

Intentions are more powerful than we assume. A parent's heart and its intentions towards the child are so pure that a higher power takes over to prevent harm. There will never be a perfect mom or a perfect child. Life will not allow it. But we'll always have plenty of perfect intentions.

"When your heart speaks, take good notes."
--Judith Campbell

when confidence is low but on its way up

Aarav was cranky every evening. We tried feeding and soothing, but these were not working. The books called it colic, but we weren't sure how to make it go away. One night when his crying did not stop for several hours, we took him to the pediatric emergency. Those were our doctor's instructions - if the baby was uncomfortable, and nothing was working, bring him in. Although it was not an emergency, it felt no less. We did not want to wait and take a chance. With premie babies, one would rather be paranoid and err on the side of caution. My only concern was the chance of him catching an infection in the emergency area. I decided to go alone, and Vineet stayed home with Aarav.

That was my first time in a pediatric emergency unit. The place was buzzing with activity even at 10pm. The female doctor on night duty was attending to another case - a small boy had broken his arm. A few feet ahead, another boy was being treated for a high fever. When it was my turn, I explained the situation to her and gave her context regarding Aarav's stay in the NICU. She did not insist on seeing the child. She suspected a version of colic or gas and prescribed a simple herbal medicine to soothe his tummy. She also gave me a list of home remedies and suggested I change the timing of his calcium supplement. She said this was normal (a word I loved those days). Talking to her calmed my nerves. The medicine also worked, and we used it a couple of times that week.

I thanked God for sending another good doctor our way. Some paediatricians play by the book - they want to see the baby before they comment, or want to be sure it is an emergency before they spend time talking to you. Typically, one is not supposed to pay consultation fees in the emergency room, so I was surprised when she took the time to do a proper consultation. I think she sensed my anxiety and the fact that Aarav was a premie. She knew that a conversation would help me. Her asking me so many questions to rule out all other possibilities made me feel my baby was okay. She told me to trust my instincts, and that boosted my confidence for the coming weeks.

The weekly trips to our original doctor continued, and each visit had an element of suspense. Aarav was weighed on a precise scale, and we would know if our care was working. We celebrated every significant rise in his weight. The standard growth charts used for full-term babies were unattainable for Aarav. My doctor drew new curves that made sense for Aarav's birth weight and told us that we should track to these instead. Some weeks his weight was off, and it took a long time for him to reach 2kg. Week 1 at home he was crying a lot, and

Week 2 he had diarrhoea after his first vaccination. In premies, vaccinations are not given at birth. They are given once the baby reaches a healthy weight, hence the extra care in avoiding infections until vaccination.

The diarrhoea episode was quite ironical. We were just getting used to the idea of him pooping once a week when suddenly he pooped five times a day. We rushed back to the doctor. We had not yet learned that it takes a few days for diarrhoea symptoms to subside. Our instincts were in training, and by the end of the first month, we were making better decisions and playing 'wait and watch' more often.

Over many such trips to doctors, I have concluded that good paediatricians focus on reducing trips to the clinic. They use email and phone generously with their patients and slowly boost the confidence of mothers to self judge the severity of the issue. They know that parents play a critical role in restoring a child's health. And they act accordingly.

where you stop counting after 3

Aarav's NICU-like care continued for the next several months. More tasks got added to the list - saline nasal drops to avoid a stuffy nose, mosquito nets, daily massages with virgin coconut oil, etc. The notebook regimen became a feature of our home, and even my sister-in-law who visited for a week learnt to fill it in.

Vineet's parents were back for a few weeks in October around Aarav's actual due date. At 2 kilograms (4.4 pounds) weight, I had started tub baths for him. He is a water baby from that first bath till today. The big day for all of us was when his weight touched 2.3 kg, and the doctor finally uttered the words that I had been craving for, "you can feed him every 3 hours unless he cries sooner". He said it as a matter of fact. I wanted to hug him tight.

Four feeds less per day! Did I mention the extra hour of sleep?! My mom-in-law and my Mom were united in their belief that Aarav should now be fed on demand, and not woken up mercilessly every three hours. After some debate, I learnt not to argue. Their wisdom was right for their kids, but my baby was different, and he will be woken up every 3 hours.

We were chanting up to the magical number of 3 kilograms (6.6 pounds) for the next several weeks. When Aarav got there, the doctor merely said - "Good job, Mom!". I was bursting with one question which I finally asked him, "Do I need to wake him up every 3 hours?"

"No. You can feed on demand. He is old enough to cry when he is hungry."
Hiding my unbounded happiness, I gave the doctor a frown that conveyed, "If I hadn't asked when were you going to tell me this sinfully delicious piece of news!"
Sometimes neonatologists forget that parents of premies actually follow instructions, and don't bend the rules.

It was celebration time at dinner that night. No wine for me, but the thought of not setting the alarm, and waking up on demand was giving me a tremendous high. I knew my son by now, and I was sure he will sleep for five hours straight, and he did. Daddy appreciated this too. Unfortunately, the NICU days had made Vineet a very light sleeper, so he had been waking up every 3 hours too.

Between the two of us, Vineet has slept more often with Aarav right through the first few years. That's because I find it hard to fall back to sleep once woken up. Vineet, on the other hand, can fall back to sleep quickly. Once I stopped breast-feeding, I slept in a separate room on many days. I could not fall back to sleep if Aarav made a sound and woke me up. It took me another two hours to get sleep, often only after I had eaten some dry fruits or had some milk. Some of my friends found it strange that we followed this routine. They're used to sleeping in the same room as their husband. Since Vineet and I both work, and know how important it is to sleep, we chose an approach that makes our family more functional. Families, where one parent takes a disproportionate share of parenting, are slowly shrinking. Not because moms don't want to take that share, but because dads wish to participate. Work-life balance is as important for dads as it is for moms.

"And here is a doctrine at which you will laugh. It seems to me, dear friend, that love is the most important thing in the world."
-- Hermann Hesse, Siddhartha

where it all finally makes sense

Our notebook was not filling up these days. Once in a while, there was an entry for something unusual like a vomit, or a question that must be asked on the next visit to the doctor. By December that year, we had permission to fly, and we took Aarav to our parents' home for a few weeks. Our son, who pooped once a week decided to poop on his maiden flight. We had a great laugh. (It wasn't easy to clean him up in the airplane bathroom, but we were happy to skip using that wretched suppository).

The baby milestones all came one by one - social smiling, turning, crawling, walking and lots of talking. They came according to his due date and not his birth date, as was the norm for premies. It was a little surreal to see how his body followed the due date calendar. The only milestone that came very early was talking. I think he was spoken to so much in the NICU, and during his 12 feeds a day that he was waiting to respond, and get us to stop! The NICU nurses spoke two South Indian languages - Kannada and Malayalam. At home, he heard three other languages - English, Hindi and Marathi. We often joked that his early gibberish was a mixture of all.

I tracked everything by his due date. This practice was so ingrained by then that when asked his age, I gave his corrected age and not his birth age. It also helped me avoid the follow on questions about why he looked smaller than other babies. Once in an elevator, an elderly neighbour asked us when he was born. I replied October while Vineet blurted out August. That moment the elevator door opened, and she had to get off, but her puzzled look said plenty, "These parents of today! Cannot even remember when their child was born!"

Vineet felt it unnecessary to explain why Aarav looked smaller and thinner as compared to other kids born in August. Soon I too stopped worrying about these silly social situations and learnt to do the same. If I was told when he was born that one day my only worry would be what age to tell others, I'd have laughed and said, "Bring it on!"

On a reflective note, if an artist was to paint my 33 years before Aarav, he would have used two or three colours. The splash of all colours appeared only after Aarav's birth. No matter how much I wanted to believe that my previous pursuits were meaningful and dictated my happiness, they didn't seem to add up. Life forced me to stop scratching the surface, and dig deeper for the real stuff.

I vividly remember one afternoon at the NICU washing area. A new cheerful mother was washing up right next to me. She asked me how my baby was doing. Her positive body language made me assume her baby was doing well too. When I asked her, she told me that her daughter had a particular neurological condition at birth, and would live for a few weeks only. She had shifted her daughter to this hospital to ensure that her baby got the best care for those few weeks. She was pumping milk and was there every day just like the rest of us. Her tremendous sense of duty as a mother had me perplexed for days. Is the heart capable of such acceptance and courage?

On another occasion, I remember having to fill some forms in the room adjoining the doctor's area. The senior-most doctor was talking to some parents. The father's voice was very anxious, almost choking, "I can take my baby to the best hospitals in the US. I am sure something can be done. Tell me if I should do that. What can I do as a father in this situation?"

"As a doctor, I can tell you, Sir, that we are doing our best, and every treatment known to the world, is available to us. I know the end is near, and I have to tell you that. But I cannot stop you if you feel otherwise. There is another baby in a similar situation in this NICU. Her father cannot afford this hospital, and every day here is a burden on her family. Yet her father is keeping her here against all odds. He is doing his duty every day. I know the situation is tough for you. Do what you believe is your duty as a father. I am doing my duty as a doctor, and trust me that if I felt you should take her elsewhere, I would tell you that."

A few babies never made it out of that NICU, and a few babies did not make it after going home. I knew those parents. I had seen their dads rushing in with freshly pumped milk, and their mothers despite the pains from delivery stitches, walking up to their babies. I had seen many, many other mothers sitting for hours in those uncomfortable chairs, baby on their chest, whispering the same mantra, singing the same songs our moms had sung for us. Every baby there was the centre of someone's life and was surrounded by love, care and tears.

Even in those days of extreme stress, there were moments of lightness. We mums chatted about our disobeying breasts or bonded over how dads have it easy, or how the formula should be improved. The first time I managed to pump 10ml (2 teaspoons), I joyfully told all the moms. They knew why I was so happy. Vineet was more like, "Is that all? no more?"

Premie dads had their own chit-chats. They would compare baby weights or exchange notes on health insurance policies. Once in a while, Dads would let their emotions show through. I remember one Dad telling Vineet that he had lost his mother last year in the same hospital. He never wanted to see that 8th floor, where her room had been allocated. A month later, when Aarav was shifted to the hospital room, we bumped into this Dad on the 11th floor. He whispered to Vineet, "They tried to give me an 8th floor room for my baby, but I waited in the NICU till we got a room on this floor."

We're all made of the same stuff on the inside - a massive ball of energy and emotions. Probably 90% of that is love. Life does not offer everyone a chance to see this ball of love and see it so visibly across so many people at the same time. Vineet and I were incredibly lucky to see that love every day.

In the past, I had worked hard towards some visible symbol of success, but now I did not feel the need to qualify or measure my work. Being with Aarav was important to me, and I respected my heart in these matters. I now value time with family more than ever before. I know that time adds up, even if it's spent doing nothing, just being around each other, with nowhere to go, and nothing to achieve. Everything does not need a counter for it to count. I try to do more of what makes me happy in this moment, for I've seen that these moments is all there is.

Money on an absolute scale lost its importance for me. It held more meaning while I was studying at Wharton, where the business school culture emphasized "more is better". After Aarav, I thought in terms of a family and not as an individual. As a family, we had enough, and I did not need to have an imbalanced life to ensure enough is always there. Both at work and at home, life seemed too short to not be myself, too short to live with half-hearted breaths, and breathing is something I had seen far too closely to know I would rather be dead than be half-alive.

I witnessed first hand how conventional spirituality does not hold up when it comes to the love and emotions that surface in difficult times. The focus on self, the path of detachment, the idea that we are alone in this world, or the mind being our path to wisdom - these principles lost meaning for me after Aarav. Living and loving from the heart, and not the mind, offer a more sure path towards wisdom and meaning. Happiness is rarely found alone. I now felt the "I" or the "me" cannot be the lead character of my story, that living for myself is a hollow and sure to fail idea. Having something to nurture gave both purpose and meaning to my everyday life. That something need not be a child, but it better be about something that's real and beyond me. Something that will nudge that heart, make it weep, laugh, jump around, and take some giant leaps of faith.

Never in a million years would I have wanted that painful NICU life for Aarav at birth. I would have hung myself upside down for nine months of pregnancy if that would have kept him inside. I feel differently when it comes to Vineet and myself. In many ways, I feel we were chosen for that experience, for that extra class with unusual lessons.

Every once in a while when I feel confused, or restless, or just incomplete in some way, I close my eyes and remember that class I took at Aarav's birth, a class filled with answers for any question life throws at me.

Thank you, Aarav.

epilogue

A short poem: Surrender

I cannot hold him right, on my first day as mommy,
"Don't fear, I'm yours forever", say the eyes of my baby.

I cannot prevent a fall, I cannot prevent those tears,
I set a bad example, never learn despite the years.
Yet my toddler repeats, "Don't fear, I'm yours forever."

I wish I could surrender to something, to someone,
as my child does to me,
as absolute, and with love that compares no one.

Can I surrender to my toddler?
"You're too young", says my mind. I know better.

To my spouse?
"You don't love the same", says my mind. I love better.

To my parents?
"Your times were different", says my mind. I learn better.

And finally - to my own Heart?
Even the thought makes my mind rant endless -
"You're crazy, you're emotional, you're penniless!"

Oh wise Heart, who knows that bliss of surrender,

forgive me for I live in my mind,
But I promise to fight back, I promise to run further,
and the day I get out, I'll be yours forever.

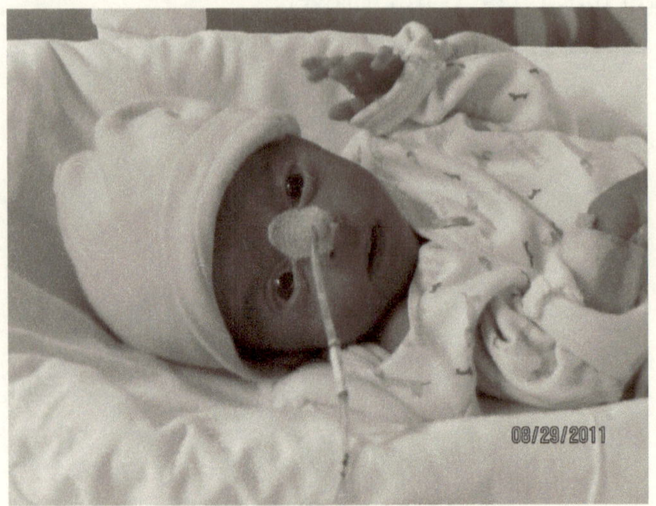

Aarav in the NICU, at 4 weeks after birth. That's when we started taking pictures.

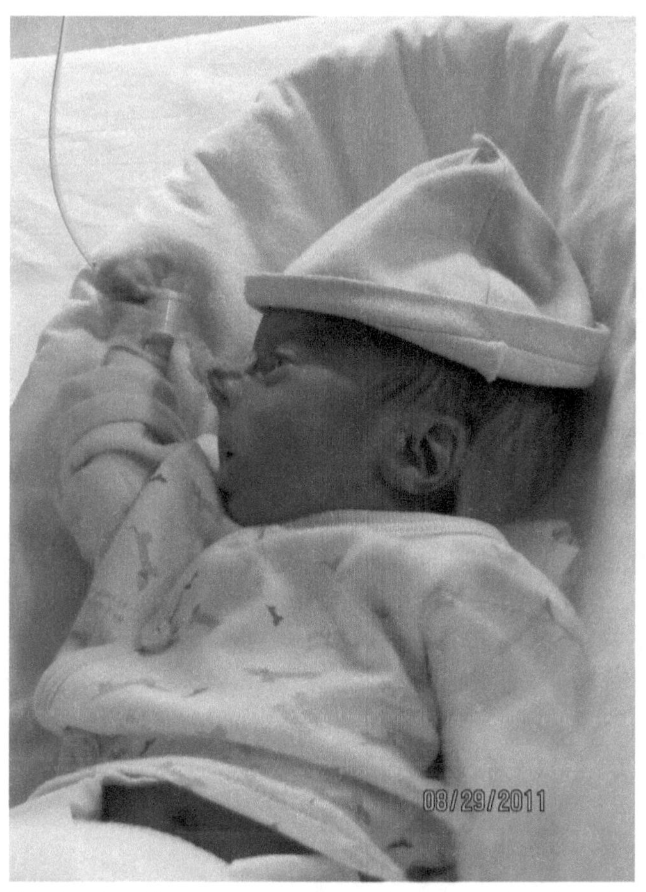

He looks like a man on a mission, with his feeding tube and all the sensors taped to his arm.

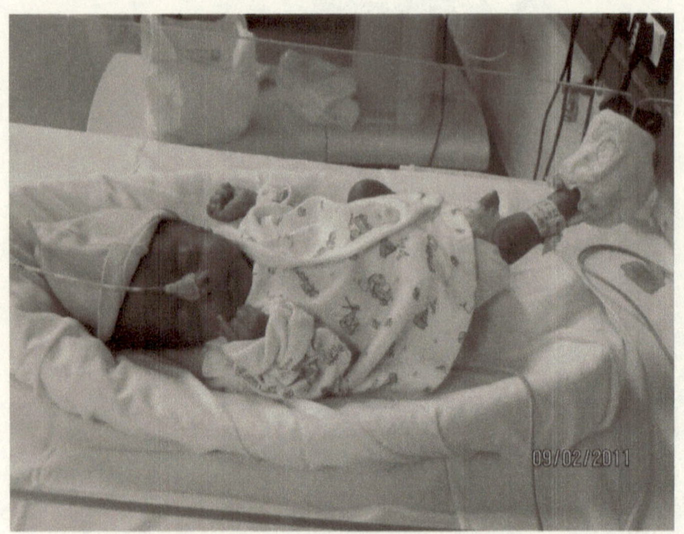

A close up of his open incubator, his oversized clothes, and his skin darkened with the UV-exposure.

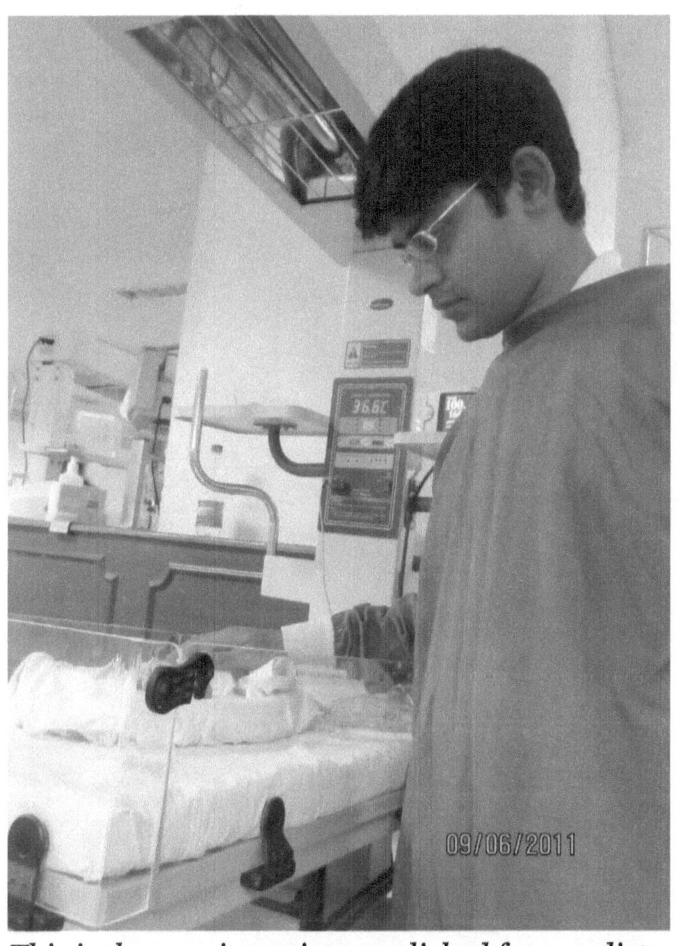

This is the previous picture, clicked from a distance. Aarav is in that little basket while Vineet pats him gently.

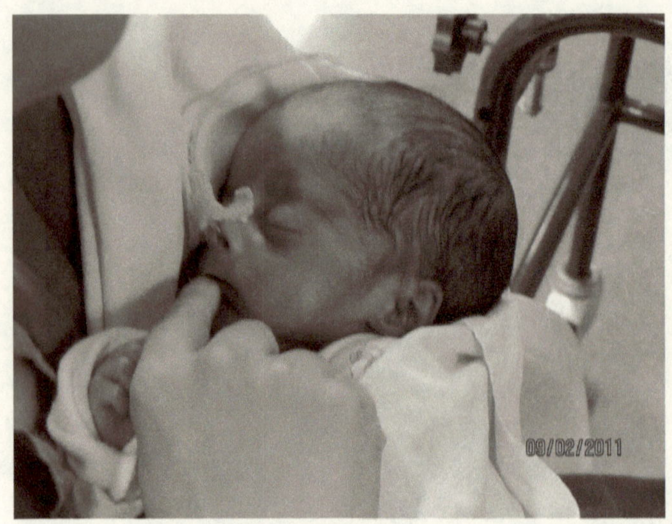

In deep sleep, while I try to nudge him to open his lips.

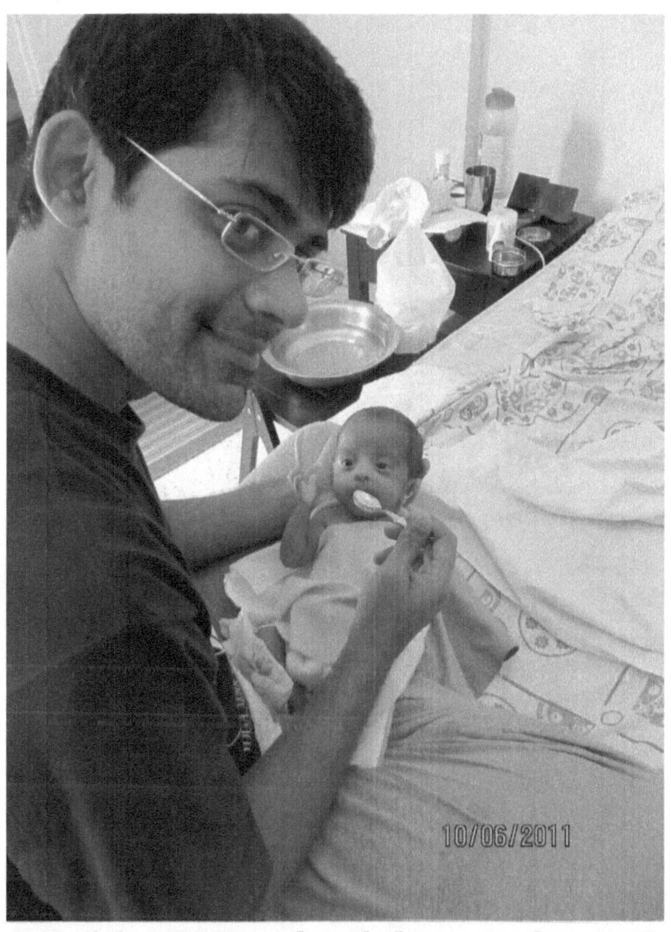

Out of the NICU, and settled into our home. Vineet's feeding him the zinc drops.

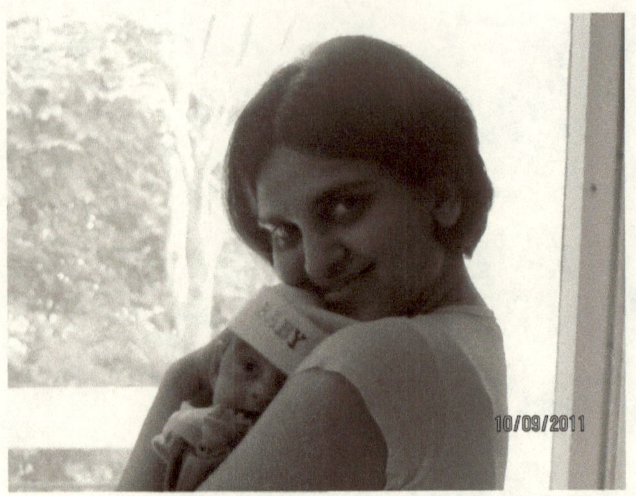

Vineet took this picture when I was showing Aarav what real sunlight feels like, for the very first time.

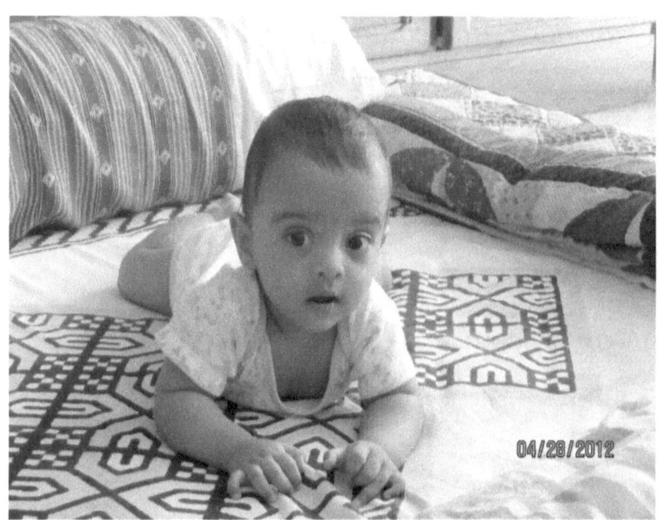

There's my big boy! Aarav at 9 months after birth.

*I hope you liked the book, and could relate to the experiences
at some level.*
I thank you for reading till the very end.

With love,
Anjali

e-mail: anjalig@gmail.com

Acknowledgements

While staying honest to the spirit of narrating this story, I
was unable to appropriately thank a few people who helped
me during my pregnancy and after.

First, my Aai and Baba. Without us having to call them, they
visited often during the bed-rest phase of my pregnancy, and
stayed for weeks on each trip. They knew we needed help,
and that we would hesitate to ask for it. They also stayed
with us for a month when Aarav was in the NICU. Aai (that's
how I refer to my mother-in-law) took care of my home, and
cheered me up with her delicious food at every meal. Baba
(my father-in-law) made several trips to the NICU to deliver
milk containers. More importantly, they allowed us to set the
rules of care, and followed them as if those rules were their
own. Their presence was always a source of comfort and
strength.

My sister-in-law Priti, for traveling to our home and staying
with me for as long as her kids' schedule permitted, and my
friend Snehal, for talking to me often, and helping me share
my emotions.